The Omega Diet

Judith Wills is one of Britain's best-known and most knowledgeable slimming and nutrition experts. The author of several bestselling books on diet, fitness and health, Judith bases her writing on sound scientific principles and up-to-date research. Her nutritional advice follows World Health Organisation and Department of Health guidelines and her life as a working mother gives her insight into the problems the average person faces when they try to adopt healthy habits.

She lives in Herefordshire with her husband and two children.

Also by Judith Wills:
Slim for Life
Take Off Ten Years in Ten Weeks
The Bodysense Diet
100 Favourite Slim and Healthy Recipes
Slim and Healthy Vegetarian
The Food Bible
Super Shape
6 Ways to Lose a Stone in 6 Weeks

First published in 2001
by HEADLINE BOOK PUBLISHING

10 9 8 7 6 5 4 3 2

ISBN 0 7472 7195 X

Designed and typeset by Ben Cracknell Studios
Printed and bound in Great Britain by Mackays of Chatham plc

HEADLINE BOOK PUBLISHING
A division of Hodder Headline
338 Euston Road
London NW1 3BH

www.headline.co.uk
www.hodderheadline.com

The Omega Diet

The Revolutionary 12-Unit Plan
for Health and Easy Weight Loss

JUDITH WILLS

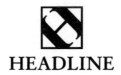

HEADLINE

Contents

The Omega Diet

I wrote *The Omega Diet* because I want you to make a fresh start.

Because I am fed up with junk food masquerading as proper, decent food and I am fed up with cranky, unbalanced and 'miracle' diets masquerading as good nutrition. And I think you are, too. I believe that very many of us feel guilty about our fast-food, mass-produced, low-nutrient meals and our surplus weight, and yet are totally confused about the right way to go.

I believe that the majority of us are looking for the diet that will help get us not only slimmer but healthier too, that offers health protection for the future, and that will help us feel good about ourselves. We want cutting-edge research, but we also want balance and truth and safe, sound nutrition.

The Omega Diet was devised and written for the sensible – yet bold – slimmer within you. For your inner voice telling you that you want to make a fresh start, but you need to be shown the way. The Omega Diet is the natural way forward both for weight loss and well-being. I believe that it is as near perfect, nutritionally, as a diet can get.

I make no apology, therefore, for the fact that it is probably a long way from the kind of diet you have been eating recently (and perhaps for much of your life). Changes are going to have to be made! When it is the well-being of your body and your health which are at stake, I am convinced that there is no point in the half-hearted approach. You either want to eat a perfect healthy diet, or you don't.

This book is for the maverick slimmer and eater. Believe me, you can do it.

And if you do, you can be assured that the advice incorporated into the Omega Diet is sound and unbiased not because of what I am, but because of what I am not.

I am not a self-styled nutritionist with a pile of vitamin pills to peddle at the end of the book. I am not a specialist who has devoted years to one tiny area of nutrition and therefore cannot see the bigger picture. I am not a consultant to a food supplement manufacturer. And I am not a disciple of any religion, sect or organisation that for reasons other than health sees fit to restrict what is good to eat.

In case you are interested in what I am, though, I am a journalist, author, researcher, mother, wife and, passionately, a lover of food and a late convert to natural well-being and health through diet. Having spent 20 years in the field of food, diet and nutrition, the last two writing, virtually single-handed, the worldwide best-selling nutritional guide *The Food Bible*, I feel thoroughly qualified to write this book.

But why Omega?

There are two reasons why this book is called *The Omega Diet*.

FIRST, 'omega' is a very important term in the field of nutrition. Omega-3 and omega-6 are the popular names of two groups of fats in the diet called 'essential fatty acids'. One of the biggest leaps forward in nutritional research in recent years has been the discovery that the right intake and balance of these types of fats has positive and probably far-reaching health benefits. There is also solid research to link a lack of certain of these fats in the modern diet with weight gain and the inability to shed weight. Up to 75% of us may be eating too little of the omega fats – or the wrong balance of them. The Omega Diet seeks to correct that balance.

While discussing the benefits of the essential fats, I have no intention, however, of giving you the impression that they are the one 'secret, magic ingredient' of a healthy diet. You will find throughout the book that all the things that are good for your body are given their due part in the Omega Diet.

SECOND, omega is the last letter of the Greek alphabet and it means 'the conclusion'. I am sure that the Omega Diet *will* conclude your weight problems, and will also provide you with a simple blueprint for healthy and enjoyable eating for the rest of your long and robust life.

Lastly, I must say again that the Omega Diet doesn't come with a promise of no effort on your part. It is a solution that will almost certainly involve you in making changes, and in becoming a realistic, as well as a sensible, slimmer. I ask you to start with an open mind and let the changes it produces in the way you look and the way you feel be the indicator of whether it is worth that effort.

In return, I will make you three promises.

One – the lifestyle changes will, within weeks or months, become second nature.

Two – if, after following the 14-day Omega Diet, you find that you have lost no weight and don't begin to feel better in yourself with at least some of the improvements listed on page 15, we will give you your money back.

Three – small improvements within weeks will become bigger improvements over the months and years if you let the Omega Diet become your last – and lasting – solution to weight loss and well-being.

Make a fresh start: you and your body deserve it.

CHAPTER 1

The Way Forward for Weight Loss

Ω

The Omega Diet provides an eating system based on just 12 food units a day, but within these units your body will get all it needs in the way of nutrients while losing weight without any form of calorie counting, weighing or calculations.

All you need to do is remember to get your 12 units a day and the diet does the rest for you.

The bonus is that you will be doing your body – and your vitality levels – both a short-term and lifelong favour if you stick with the Omega Units eating system.

On pages 14–15 you will find two checklists adding up to over 25 ways in which your body and your health may benefit by eating the Omega way. Turn to it now and see how many you would like to achieve. If you need motivation, this is surely it.

But first, this chapter sets out to answer your questions on exactly why we become overweight or obese and what slimming methods really work, and to explain the most important links between diet and health. Armed with this information, it will be easy to understand the more detailed Omega Diet advice that follows.

The modern curse of obesity

There is no doubt that obesity is becoming one of the most important health problems of our age. In the UK alone, the number of obese people has more than doubled in the past 20 years, according to the International Obesity Task Force. Now 20% of women and 17% of men have a body mass index (the standard index by which weight is measured) over 30, which indicates a health risk.

And approximately 50% of women and 40% of men have a body mass index over the desirable average of 20–25. In truth, the population has been getting slowly larger and larger since the 1950s. As time goes on, unless something is done about it, no doubt these men and women with BMIs over 25 will also join the ranks of the seriously obese. In the USA, the picture is the same. For every person following a healthy diet there, a dozen more are eating themselves into an early grave.

Worldwide, the signs are that the same will eventually happen almost everywhere. Countries which have previously had a good record for weight control and obesity-linked diseases are now succumbing, and national average weights are rising fast, along with related illnesses such as heart disease and diabetes.

For the first time in the history of the world, we now have more overweight people than underfed people – and that is official.

Back in the UK, there is a line, frequently repeated in the media, that we are actually consuming fewer calories than we did 20 years ago, but this is a fallacy. The UK Ministry of Agriculture puts out figures every three months for household consumption of food – but the key word here is *household*. The figures take no account of the very many calories consumed outside the home in takeaways, sandwich bars, pubs, clubs, cafes, restaurants and so on. These figures also exclude all the drinks consumed outside the home, as well as the calories from alcohol consumed inside it.

My estimate is that if anyone did a proper survey of all the calories consumed from whatever source by individuals in the UK, the average would show that, indeed, we are consuming far more calories than ever before.

The pundits who fall for the 'we're eating fewer calories' argument say that lack of activity is the real cause of our obesity and that all we need to do is take more exercise and the problem will be solved. Of course, we need to take more exercise, and this will *help* to solve the problem – but the basic truth is that if we want to lose weight, collectively and individually, we need to address the problem of what we are eating.

Doing it collectively is, I think, the key. It is very hard to battle single-handed with a change of diet when all around you are content to carry on as before.

Why we overeat

And here, I'm afraid, we must look at the reasons behind the massive increase in calorie consumption that has occurred in the past few decades. It can be summed up in one word: profit. Big – no, not big – huge, gigantic companies are making lots and lots of profit out of our habit of eating and drinking more than we need.

It is in the interests of food growers, producers, retailers and some sections of the advertising industry and the media who are in work because of food advertising to keep us eating and drinking more food and drink than is necessary – or healthy. And preferably the kind of food with the highest profit margins, which means commercial, processed food and drink.

We eat because we are persuaded to eat. The more we consume, the greater the profit. And, after decades of practice, the food industry and its sideshoots grow ever more clever with their powers of persuasion. They know exactly how to make us buy. Who hasn't ever walked into a supermarket to buy certain items, and walked out with at least some things they didn't intend to get or didn't even want? Who hasn't ever walked into a supermarket and bought multipacks when one small pack would have sufficed? Who hasn't ever gone to a restaurant and ordered a dessert when it wasn't really needed – but because the description in the menu was enticing? Who hasn't ever sat in front of the TV, having just eaten supper, seen an advert for chocolate, and gone searching in the larder for some?

If we could get back to eating because we are hungry, or need the nutrition in what we eat, then we wouldn't have an obesity problem at all. And we would save lots and lots of money.

Let the Omega Diet work for you

The Omega Diet will work for you only if you recognise that you have been persuaded – not to say press-ganged – into buying and eating what you don't really want and certainly don't need. It will work if you accept that you need to make a fresh start. It will work if you accept that a healthy body is more important than a learned taste for the wrong types of food. And it will work if you know that good, nutritious food isn't the same as brightly packaged, slickly sold food.

The Omega Diet is the diet for people with minds of their own. At first you may need to be strong to stick with it but if enough people get the message, big business may have to do some fairly drastic rethinking about the food they sell.

And before you ask, no, I am not against supermarket shopping as a whole. I shop in supermarkets but I have learnt to buy only what I want to buy for what I hope are the right reasons. I have weaned myself out of the multipack, ready-meal mentality, even though I have two children and want quick meals.

What I do know is that if you fill your shopping trolley with too many highly processed foods, you will get overweight and you will not be providing your body with the nutrients it needs for good health.

Malnourished though overweight

There is much documentation on the link between a highly refined diet and overweight. A diet high in saturated fats, trans (commercially hardened) fats and refined sugar leads to overeating.

There is some research to indicate that this is partly because the body recognises that it isn't getting good nutrition. In effect the modern refined diet is starving the body of nutrients, so we eat more food instinctively, trying to get those missing nutrients. In other words, people on the typical Western high-fat, high-sugar diet are suffering from malnutrition, while getting fatter and fatter!

It has been shown that extra calories are easy to take in when you eat refined foods – they just slip down. Refined foods that combine both fat and sugar are the worst culprits. Calories in drink do the same.

As you read through the chapters ahead you will find more and more evidence linking good wholesome food with the body's ability to maintain a reasonable weight. By concentrating on good Omega foods, hunger need never be a problem.

But some of you will be thinking, why, anyway, does overweight matter so much? Well, to many of us it matters because we don't like the way it looks or feels, or the way it makes US feel – and I think that is fair enough.

Even more important, gross overweight or obesity is linked absolutely with ill health and a shortened lifespan, in many ways. Heart disease, atherosclerosis, stroke, diabetes, arthritis, for instance. There's a probable link with some forms of cancer, infertility, risks in pregnancy and childbirth, high blood pressure and more.

People get symptoms of coronary heart disease (CHD) seven years earlier, on average, if they are obese.

Overweight is not healthy, is not usually attractive and is not the image that most of us want to present. (Neither, it has to be said, is underweight – we are looking for a reasonable bodyweight here, not thinness.)

So which diet for you?

If you are not sure whether you need to lose weight, or how much you need to lose, turn to Appendix 1.

If you do need to lose weight, the next question is 'How?'

A plethora of different dieting methods over the past few years has confused rather than enlightened us.

Most of the famous diets have relied upon selling a single 'new' idea' (fat free or high protein or carb free or sugar free or food combining, for example), but at the end of the day most of them don't work because of any amazing scientific breakthrough principle involved, but because they reduce one's total calorie intake.

Many are not healthy ways to lose weight because they tend to 'talk up' one particular food type at the expense of all others, creating an unbalanced and possibly dangerous diet. Too much of one nutrient (however good it may be in normal quantities) and too little of others is not good nutrition or good dieting.

The revived popularity of the high-protein diet is a good example – a high-protein intake being positively harmful for many people. Too much animal protein in the diet can cause serious kidney problems, and may increase the risk of osteoporosis and high blood pressure.

Other popular diets alter the *way* in which you are allowed to consume food types, which may also be harmful. For instance, we have the food combining (Hay) system, which tells you not to eat protein and carbohydrate at the same meal and also encourages you to eat nothing but fruit before lunchtime. This can play havoc with your blood sugar levels, and cause negative physical and mental symptoms, as well as being pointless.

In between all these trendy diets good old 'calorie counting' has always been there. The logic goes something like this: arm yourself with a book containing the calorie values of all food and drink, restrict yourself to a set number of calories a day (usually somewhere between 1,000 and 1,500) and you can make it up as you go along, as long as you stick to your calorie total.

This looks, at first, like a jolly good idea. Advocates say it prevents faddy eating, gives variety and allows you to pick foods you enjoy, while guaranteeing weight loss. In theory, this is true; but in practice, daily calorie counting is not as foolproof as it looks.

First, it is tedious because in order to get an accurate tally of your calorie intake you need to weigh and measure everything that you eat and drink and become an avid label reader if buying commercial foods. So people end up just guessing their portions and stop losing weight. Secondly, if you do it right it may guarantee weight loss, but not necessarily good health, because you may choose foods that don't add up to a balanced or healthy diet. Certainly, most people who are overweight have been eating low-nutrient or unbalanced-nutrient meals – and carrying on eating the same foods, but in a smaller quantity, is not a recipe for health or long-term slimness. And thirdly, hunger is often a problem on a calorie-counting diet because, again, low-calorie processed foods are not offering the body the sustenance it needs.

So what's wrong with low-fat dieting?

Lastly, let's take a slightly longer look at the one great popular diet of the 1980s and 1990s – the low-fat diet. This is everyone's idea of the ultimate healthy way to eat. Kill all the fat! Up the carbs! And until quite recently most experts seemed to agree that this was, indeed, the ideal way to eat and to diet. Fat – not only a cause of heart disease, but also the most fattening thing you can eat, and therefore the obvious thing to give up. Carbs – filling, lower in calories and full of fibre. The obvious thing to step up!

Partially, this still holds true. But it seems now that the experts got it wrong about fat. A very low-fat diet can be BAD for you, not good. They also got other things wrong about fat, all of which you will discover in the next chapter.

The diet experts have also learnt, through human experiments, that the high-carb, low-fat diet isn't always a very good way of losing weight: humans can get or stay fat on a high-carb diet, even without the fat. It's also known now that a very low-fat diet isn't as hunger-satisfying as other diets.

What about a high-fat diet, then – of which there are more than one about at the moment? Sorry – no good either. High-fat diets have to restrict something, otherwise they would be high in calories, so they usually restrict carbohydrates to a very, very low level. This imbalance is no good for health – low-carb diets can cause digestive disorders and other worrying symptoms. High-fat diets are also usually much too high in animal protein, which can cause serious problems, as we've already discussed above.

But before you get depressed about all these dieting methods that don't work for many people, or are dangerous to health, let me cheer you up. You don't need to be a Harvard scientist or an Emeritus Professor of Nutrition (neither of which I am) to realise that there has got to be a way of losing weight that is both safe and effective, and not too much hassle.

The natural way to slim

And of course, there is. I devised the Omega Diet to be as perfect a diet as I could make it. I wanted a diet that fulfilled all the healthy eating criteria about which you will learn more in the pages that follow. I wanted a diet that offered not just basic nutritional health but 'added nutritional value' where possible – health protection on a plate, if you like.

I wanted it to be effective – so, of course, it will advocate cutting down the amount of calories you are consuming on a regular basis. And it had to be simple to follow without involving any weighing of portions, or much more than using a spoon or cup for any measurements (the exception being some of the recipes at the back of the book –

but I don't think anyone expects recipes to come weighing- and measuring-free).

I also wanted it to be based on foods that are good to eat. And this is where some of you may at first disagree. If you've been brought up on a highly refined diet, the Omega Diet may take some getting used to because it is, for the most part, based on natural foods.

The Omega Diet is a grown-up diet for people who care about their bodies and want to put them first.

How the Omega Diet works

What I have done is work out an eating system that breaks the diet down into 12 units, called Omega Units. To lose weight, all you have to do each day is have one of each of the 12 units (combined as and when you like, by and large) and you will have perfect nutrition as well – all the fat, protein, carbs, vitamins, minerals, fibre and so on that your body needs (unless you have special needs, discussed in Chapter 8), as well as all the newer ingredients that nutritionists and scientists are discovering within our natural foods which can help both health and weight control.

The 12 units are as follows:

Protein Unit	Green Unit
Oil Unit	Flame Unit
Nut Unit	Pulse Unit
Seed Unit	Quality Carb Unit
C-Fruit Unit	Calcium Unit
Fruit 2 Unit	Water Unit

You also have many unlimited items to add variety and palatability. The Omega Units are discussed in more detail in chapters 2 to 5 and the Omega system is explained in detail in Chapters 6, 7 and 8. But to reassure you, here you can see at a glance how the Omega system provides all the nutrients within these 12 units. In later weeks, you can add extra items to your diet, for long-term slimming or weight maintenance as explained in Chapter 8.

Nutrients provided by Omega Units

Protein: Found in greatest quantities in the Protein, Calcium and Pulse Units and also in the Nut and Seed Units.

Carbohydrate: Found in greatest quantity in the Quality Carb Unit but also in the C-Fruit and Fruit-2 Units, the Flame and Green Units and the Pulse Unit.

Fat: Found in greatest quantities in the Fat Unit but also in the Protein, Nut and Seed units, as well as in other units in small quantities.

Fibre: Found in greatest quantities in the Pulse, Quality Carb, the two fruit units and Flame and Green Units, but also in the Nut and Seed Units.

Vitamin C: Found in greatest quantities in the two fruit units and the Flame and Green Units.

Vitamin B group: Found in most units, including the Quality Carb, Pulse, Nut, Seed, Protein Units.

Vitamin E: Found in greatest quantities in the Fat, Protein, Pulse, Nut, Seed, and Quality Carb Units.

Vitamin A: Found in greatest quantities in the Calcium, Fruit-2, Flame and Green Units.

Vitamin D: Found mostly in the Protein Unit.

Iron: Found in greatest quantities in the Quality Carb, Pulse, Nut, Seed, Green and Protein Units.

Calcium: Found in greatest quantities in the Calcium Unit, but also in the Protein, Nut, Seed and Green Units.

Zinc: Found in greatest quantities in the Protein, Quality Carb, Pulse, Nut and Seed Units.

Selenium: Found in greatest quantities in the Nut, Seed, Pulse, Protein and Quality Carb Units.

Magnesium: Found in greatest quantities in the Nut, Seed, Quality Carb, Green and Water Units.

Eating the Omega way not only reduces calories, but also has extra slimming bonuses: I have used the latest food research to ensure that your body gets all the help it can. For instance, pulses help regulate blood sugar to avoid hunger pangs. Omega-3 oils may help to metabolise food, while food with a low glycaemic index may help to burn calories quicker, and so on.

Good health for life

The same foods that will get and keep you slim for the rest of your life can also help you to get and stay healthy, and generally feel good. Even better, they can help prevent disease and degeneration.

This is just such a good fact to know because many people have a job motivating themselves to keep on with a calorie-reduced diet. If your short-term well-being and your long-term health aren't motivation enough – I can't think of anything better.

What you will read in the pages ahead are not half-truths or blatant exaggerations. The information is based on sound scientific research, overviews and consensus of opinion. Where there is any doubt, I will say so.

Bearing that in mind, I am going to give you two lists to run through. Here's List One, starting from the top:

Do you suffer from any of these?

Headaches	Joint aches and pains
Dizziness	Painful neck glands
Dull eyes	Frequent infections
Dry skin	Indigestion
Dull, dry hair	Flatulence
Bleeding gums	Bloating of the stomach
Tooth decay	Constipation
Tiredness	PMS
Insomnia	Hot flushes
Depression	

All of these symptoms or disorders may be greatly eased or even prevented or cured completely by the Omega Diet.

Now here's List Two:

Would you like to be at lower risk of getting any of these?

High blood pressure	Osteoarthritis
Coronary heart disease	Rheumatoid arthritis
Atherosclerosis	Cancer of the bowel
Stroke	Alzheimer's disease
Diabetes type 2	Osteoporosis

All these conditions and diseases of the 21st century may be either helped, prevented or even cured by the Omega Diet.

The Omega Diet promise

The Omega Diet can have you beginning to feel better in yourself, with symptoms from List One beginning to ease, after days or weeks. And it can give you long-term health protection from the ailments in List Two: the risk of major diseases decreases with each month and year that you stay with the system. AND don't forget – it can get you slim!

This may seem a tall order for a simple, straightforward, inexpensive diet. It may sound too good to be true that you can do this without any miracle foods or new-fangled ingredients or strange-sounding supplements or odd ways of combining foods. I repeat there are no magic pills offered in the diet, other than the magic pill of good nutrition itself. What you see is what you get, and is all explained in what I hope is plain English, with no twisting of the truth in order to make the ideas seem more amazing or exciting than they really are.

I don't see the point in that – because the truth is amazing enough. And in the chapters ahead you will learn more about what particular health benefits can be gained from each food group in the Omega system.

My promise is that if you follow the system it will work, and you will feel good without worrying about what makes a healthy diet, without worrying about calorie or fat counting. Quite simply, this is the easiest way of losing pounds and eating right that's ever been devised. All it needs now is for *you* to be prepared to take the step . . . and I believe that the following chapters will give you all the encouragement you need.

CHAPTER 2

Oils for Health

Since the 1980s, both dieters and health-watchers have been led to believe that fat is 'bad'. Many of us have therefore resolutely followed a fat-free or low-fat path whenever possible. For many people, fat avoidance has become an obsession – and one which continues unabated today. For all that time, I have resolutely refused to join the low-fat lobby.

Not only is a very low-fat diet unpalatable, but I have always instinctively felt – even when the research wasn't there to back up my feelings – that as fat was a natural part of many of our most basic foods, it couldn't possibly be as bad for us as was made out.

I knew that to try to avoid fat at all costs wasn't a balanced or healthy way to eat. And I knew that some of nature's most glorious foods, such as olive oil, fish, nuts, seeds and avocados, were high in fat.

Very many years ago, the first proof began to come through that certain types of fat were actually good for the health and not harmful. We have long known that the Mediterranean diet produces longevity. Now we are beginning to find out the scientific answers as to why and how.

There is a long way to go, but we have found out enough new evidence to turn on its head the idea of the low-fat diet as the right way to slimness and health.

We also now know that the experts did almost certainly get one huge area of advice on fat consumption wrong.

Throughout the 1990s, the advice was not just to cut fat intake, but to replace the saturated fats (found mostly in animal and dairy produce) with polyunsaturated oils such as corn and sunflower oil. This advice was taken on board in a huge way throughout the Western world.

But occasionally studies seemed to disprove the theory that poly-unsaturates were the answer to healthy fat consumption. One famous trial in Wales appeared to show that eating good old-fashioned butter resulted in less incidence of heart disease than consuming sunflower margarine.

17

More evidence was amassed to show that people who ate high amounts of corn and sunflower oils and low amounts of saturated fat had just as high a death rate as those who did the opposite – even though the rates of death from heart disease were lower in the former group. They just died from other things, especially increased rates of cancer.

Meanwhile, in the Western world other ills were on the increase – diabetes, arthritis, Alzheimer's, asthma and depression, for example.

Amazingly, it has now been found that far from helping our general health, our huge intake of 'modern' oils, such as corn and sunflower oil, may actually be one of the main problems! The rest of this chapter is devoted to helping you to eat the right kind of fats in the right balance and the right quantities both for health and for help with slimming.

Saturated fat: still on the 'go easy' list

The basic advice on consumption of saturated fat in the diet for most of us hasn't changed. A high intake of saturates – found in greatest quantities in full-fat dairy produce, fatty cuts of meat, meat and poultry skin and eggs – is still compellingly linked with heart disease, stroke and related problems, or precursors such as obesity and high blood pressure.

It is still extremely easy in the West (and more common in the rest of the world) to consume far too much saturated fat because we eat so much commercial food, such as cakes, pastries, pies, biscuits, desserts, packet goods, takeaways such as burgers, hot dogs, meat and cheese pizzas, and so on. All of these are often high in saturates. We also eat a diet high in cheese, cream, eggs, fried foods, pastry, butter and fatty meat at home, with our main daily meals often out of balance in favour of high-saturate foods. Added to that, we eat too much – and the big portions we give ourselves add to the total of saturated fat that we eat.

The World Health Organisation suggests a limit of 10% of our total calorie intake on saturated fat, yet many of us eat twice that much. The Omega Diet provides less than 5% of its calories as saturated or their 'cousins', trans fats.

Trans fats: the recent culprits

Many of us have now heard of trans fats. These fats start out before the manufacturing process as polyunsaturated fats, but are altered and hardened during the processing stages to become trans fats – no longer unsaturated, but saturated and similar in their effects on our bodies to other saturates.

Many experts believe that trans fats are actually worse for us than saturated fats. Indeed, one study last year showed that the effect trans fats have on the ratio of 'bad to good' cholesterol may be twice as bad as that of saturated fat. And at least saturates such as butter and lard are 'natural', unadulterated foods, whereas trans fats are not. So it seems highly probable that the first fats to cut out of your diet are trans fats.

Sadly, most of the highly processed foods that don't contain saturates (and are often labelled as 'low in saturates') are actually high in trans fats. Many margarines, and lots of biscuits, cakes and other baked goods are high in trans fats.

The *US Nurses Study* found that nurses who ate hydrogenated margarines regularly were 50% more likely to contract heart disease than nurses who didn't.

The main lines on saturates and trans

Here's what we know so far about the 'bad' fats.

Ω Goods that are high in either saturates or trans fats tend also to be low on other natural nutrients such as dietary fibre, naturally occurring vitamins, and so on.

Ω Saturates may also negate the effects of the 'good' fats, about which we will talk in a page or two.

So the first thing the Omega Diet does is to drastically reduce your intake of both saturated fats and trans fats to less than 5% of your total calorie intake.

Polyunsaturated fats: a diverse family

Back in the 1980s when the idea that saturated fats were 'bad for you' became common knowledge, we became very familiar with poly-unsaturated fats. As you'll recall, these fats are found in high quantities in oils extracted from plants such as corn, sunflower and safflower. They were touted as 'good for you', because they didn't have a negative effect on blood lipids, and actually had a positive effect in lowering LDL cholesterol (the kind that is bad for you) in the blood – thus helping to prevent coronary heart disease and stroke.

Much research backed this theory up, so we embarked upon a 20-year love affair with the stuff – cooking with sunflower oil, spreading sunflower-based margarines on our bread instead of butter, and generally buying anything with the word 'polyunsaturated' printed on the pack, all the while feeling very virtuous and healthy.

What now? The main theory remains true, that polyunsaturates lower 'bad' LDL blood cholesterol. BUT we now know that this is only one side of the coin.

Before I can proceed with this story, you need to know a bit about the family tree of the polyunsaturates, because the differences between them are crucial.

The group of fatty acids known as polyunsaturates can be divided into two 'families' – the N6 group (the omega-6s) and the N3 group (the omega-3s).

All the polyunsaturated oils that we have been encouraged to use in our diets are the ones that contain a much higher proportion of the omega-6 types of fatty acid than of the omega-3s. These include safflower oil, sunflower oil and corn oil.

Here I should point out that fat extracted from any plant won't just contain ONE type of fatty acid. It will contain not only polyunsaturates – maybe from both omega-6s and omega-3s – but also a certain amount of the other fats, mono-unsaturates and saturates. It is impossible to find any oil from a natural source which isn't a combination of more than one type of fatty acid.

For example, sunflower oil is typical of what we think of as a 'polyunsaturated' oil. In fact, it contains 12% of saturates and 20% of mono-

unsaturates. But its dominant oil is polyunsaturated and within this polyunsaturated family, approximately 67.5% is composed of omega-6s, and 0.75% is made up of omega-3s. Even a so-called 'saturated fat' like butter contains approximately 3.5% polyunsaturates and 25% mono-unsaturates.

The main reason that the polyunsaturates which are most popular with the food industry are high in omega-6s and low in omega-3s is simple: the foods which are a good source of omega-3s are much less easy, or more expensive, to produce commercially, and there are fewer of them. These include linseed oil, walnut oil and fish oils. And to be fair, it is only in recent years that anyone has even thought to question the source of the 'good for you' polyunsaturates. So, without any compelling reason to get our polyunsaturates from the omega-3 group, there has been no cause for change.

But now we have a compelling reason!
In fact, we have TWO.

Here are the facts that will convince you that it is time to take a new look at polyunsaturated fats.

FACT ONE: A typical Western diet high in omega-6 polyunsaturates may cause more health problems than it cures. It is now known that a diet high in omega-6s is linked with an increased risk of cancer and increased rate of tumour growth.

It is also known that the original advice to eat polyunsaturates to lower LDL blood cholesterol was naive. Not only do most leading experts now agree that lowering of LDL cholesterol is probably by no means the most important factor in beating heart disease, but we now know that our high omega-6 diet actually increases the oxidation of the LDL cholesterol. This is dangerous, as oxidised cholesterol is then deposited on the arterial walls, by which it becomes a major factor in increased risk of atherosclerosis, stroke and heart disease.

Polyunsaturates are highly prone to oxidation (when fat goes rancid, it is oxidised but your oil will not necessarily taste or smell rancid even if it is oxidised). Heat, light and exposure to oxygen will encourage this effect. In other words, the omega-6 oils (and, indeed, the omega-3 oils) stored in warm, light conditions and in the presence of oxygen (such as in the typical kitchen) will soon oxidise. Cooking at high temperatures means that all the 'good effect' of the oil in lowering LDL cholesterol is cancelled out because you are oxidising the oil. As most of us who buy corn, safflower and sunflower oil use it for cooking, this is a big problem.

A high intake of omega-6 oils also blocks the good work of the omega-3 oils, which brings me on to . . .

FACT TWO: It is more important to get the omega-3s and omega-6s in the right balance within your diet – while cutting down on the saturated fat that you eat – than it is to increase the total amount of poly-unsaturates in your diet.

Much research in the past 20 years or more has been done on the relationship between a healthy heart and the omega-3s (see panel on page 25), but now much more work is being done in other areas, and we are discovering that the omega-3 oils may have wide-ranging health benefits.

Here are just some of the recent findings:

Ω *Cancer prevention* Omega-3 fatty acids slow down the growth of tumours in rats considerably, and all the evidence so far leads to the fact that this is also true in humans, although more work needs to be done. Omega-3s also appear to help prevent new tumours from starting and help to prevent them from spreading. Omega-3s boost our immune system, which may help pre-cancerous cells from developing and have been shown to help fight infection on a general level.

Ω *Arthritis* Adequate intake of the omega-3 fats EPA and DHA (see panel on page 25) have been clearly shown to improve the symptoms of rheumatoid arthritis (using supplements). Omega-3s may also help other inflammatory diseases, such as Crohn's disease, asthma and even gingivitis, although the research is less clear.

Ω *Diabetes* Omega-3s, particularly DHA, are linked with an improvement in insulin sensitivity, and a high ratio of omega-3s to omega-6s in the diet is linked with improved glycaemic control, both of which are important factors in non-insulin-dependent diabetes. Diabetes is discussed in more detail in Chapters 4 and 5.

Ω *Depression* A balanced ratio and adequate intake of omega-6s and omega-3s may help to prevent or relieve depression and improve mood and behaviour.

Ω *Brain power* It was an 'old wives' tale' that fish was good for the brain – now it seems that oily fish, at least, may well be so! There is encouraging research to show that high consumption of EPA and DHA can lead to lower risk of Alzheimer's disease, and a lack of essential fatty acids in the diet is also linked with dyslexia, attention deficit disorder, dyspraxia (clumsy child syndrome) and other behavioural problems in children.

Ω *Early development* The omega fats are now known to be particularly important for the healthy brain development of babies both in the womb and early in life, and therefore pregnant and breast-feeding women should ensure adequate intakes.

Ω *Skin complaints* Deficiency in omega-3s may also be linked with skin complaints such as psoriasis or general dry, flaky or itchy skin conditions.

However, we all need some omega-6 fats in our diet. Indeed, the 'parent' fatty acid of the omega-6 group, linoleic acid, is called an 'essential fatty acid' because our bodies can't manufacture it and we must get it through our diet. The only other 'essential fatty acid' (EFA) is linolenic acid, the 'parent' of the omega-3 group, about which we talk more in the panel on page 25.

The omega-6s and omega-3s have much everyday hard work to do within our bodies, helping to produce hormones for good health and helping us in many other ways, including wound healing, liver and kidney function, healthy skin, reproduction and good growth, healthy hair and a healthy nervous system. These roles of the essential fatty acids have been known for some time. But the importance of the *balance* of intake of the two is a newer area of research.

It now seems that the 'good work' of the omega-3s can be blocked by over-consumption of the omega-6s (and of the saturated and trans fats) which, as we saw earlier in the chapter, is a problem that probably applies to most of us eating the typical Western diet.

Some estimates say that we may have been eating as much as 20 times more omega-6 than omega-3, other estimates put it lower at seven times as much, which is still too high. What we need to do is increase the omega-3s in our diet and decrease the omega-6s until a correct balance is restored, while not increasing the overall level of polyunsaturates at all.

The Omega Diet will provide you with a maximum ratio of 4:1 and a minimum ratio of 2:1, and the total amount of poyunsaturates in the diet is approximately 10%. This total percentage is about the same as a typical Western diet – it is the *balance* we are going to alter.

The link between the kind of fats that you eat and your weight

Apart from the benefits described above, the omega-3 fats almost certainly have an important role to play in slimming and weight maintenance as well.

Omega-3s seem to help regulate the body's blood sugar levels by helping to increase insulin sensitivity. This means that hunger can be kept at bay (for more on blood sugars see Chapters 4 and 5) – and in the long term it also means less risk of both diabetes and obesity. Again, a low omega-6 to omega-3 ratio may be the key factor here. Interestingly, many experts reckon that at least 25% of adults in the Western world are insulin resistant. If you have had trouble losing weight on a regular, high-carbohydrate, low-fat diet, a diet high in omega-3s may well be your answer.

Even more interesting is that a diet high in the omega-6 fats, when fed to mice who are also getting a low intake of omega-3s, causes the mice to gain as much weight as a diet high in saturated fats, whereas a diet high in omega-3s causes them to lose weight.

Of course, mice and men are not the same – but often the results of experiments carried out on rodents can be replicated in humans. Initial research shows that indeed this may be the case.

For instance, Udo Erasmus, the world-famous expert on oils in nutrition, says that omega-3s work by increasing our metabolic rate so that more fat and glucose are burned and less deposited as body fat. He

The family of omega-3s

The omega-3 family of polyunsaturates includes several related fatty acids. At the 'head' of the family is *alpha-linolenic acid*, called an 'essential fatty acid' because it cannot be made in our bodies so we need to get it through our diet. The foods highest in this (while also being low or lowish in omega-6s) are linseed oil and linseeds, walnut oil and rapeseed oil, but it is also present in good amounts in green vegetables, and is present in lamb and game.

Further on down the group come two very interesting fatty acids, DHA and EPA. Most medical research to date on the omega-3 group has been done using DHA and EPA. If our bodies are working well and our diet is in balance, DHA and EPA can be made in the body from alpha-linolenic acid, though you need to eat a lot more alpha-linolenic acid to get the same amount of DHA and EPA.

But it is possible – and probably preferable – to get DHA and EPA direct from the diet, and just about the only natural sources of these fatty acids in the diet are fish and fish oils. A regular intake of these oils is linked incontrovertibly with lowered blood lipid (fat) levels, and thus a lowered risk of atherosclerosis, lowered blood pressure in people with high blood pressure, and a reduction in the tendency of the blood to clot, and thus the prevention of cardiovascular diseases.

It seems that the optimum diet for health contains adequate omega-3s in the form of both alpha-linolenic acid, DHA and EPA.

A list of the DHA and EPA contents of various types of fish appears under Unit One on page 31.

also says that omega-3s increase our energy levels and encourage us to take more exercise, which in turn builds more lean tissue (muscle), which in turn increases our metabolic rate even more, as muscle cells are the most metabolically active in our bodies.

More work needs to be done on the whole topic before we can be sure of the facts. Meanwhile, as a high omega-3 diet has so many other advantages, and, apparently, no known disadvantages, it is surely worth going down the omega-3 route if you are overweight.

Getting the right balance of omega fats into your diet

I won't fudge. In order to achieve a ratio of no more than four times as much omega-6 as omega-3, fairly sweeping changes to the typical Western diet have to be made. This is because although both omega-6s and omega-3s are present in most plant foods, the ratio of omega-6 is much higher in all the oils that we typically consume in greatest quantities. For example, the polyunsaturated fat in safflower oil is almost 100% omega-6s, giving an omega-6 to omega-3 ratio of over 200:1! You need to make a quite determined effort to avoid the omega-6s in most situations in order to make more 'room' for the higher omega-3 oils.

A glance at the omega chart opposite will show you the extent of the problem. Only linseeds and linseed oil actually contain more omega-3s than omega-6s; with the exception of some game meats such as rabbit and quail, which are very low in fat anyway and thus won't be anything other than a very minor source of omega-3s in the diet. And only rapeseed oil and pumpkin seeds contain an omega-6 to omega-3 ratio of less than 4:1.

The oily fishes described on page 31 will make a significant contribution to your omega-3 intake in the form of EPA and DHA, but even they also contain some omega-6 fats. So making informed choices in the types of fatty food that you eat is extremely important.

The Omega Diet aims to provide you with the correct balance of omega oils. Appendix 2 on page 175 charts out, as exactly as possible, the average amount of the different fats the 14-day diet will provide you with, and translates these into percentages of your total diet, for those of you who are interested in the detail.

Obviously, it is not possible to be accurate to the last gram, not least because there is a degree of choice on the 14-day diet and a great deal of choice afterwards, but also because amounts in fresh foods do vary according to season, age of produce, storage conditions, and so on. But you can be assured that if you follow the Omega Diet and its guidelines for long-term eating, you will be improving your balance of polyunsaturated fats to an optimum degree. The Omega Diet will also help you consume oils of optimum quality and nutritional benefit – for instance, ensuring that oxidisation is kept at a minimum and that vitamin and mineral content is maximised.

Omega fatty acid content of foods
(in g per 100g)†

Omega-6s		Omega-3s*	
Safflower oil	74	Linseed oil	53
Grapeseed oil	68	Linseeds	14
Sunflower oil	63	Walnut oil	11.5
Walnut oil	58	Rapeseed oil	9.5
Soya oil	51	Soya oil	7
		Pumpkin seeds	7**
Corn oil	50	Walnuts	5.5
Sesame oil	43	Quail	2.5
Polyunsaturated		Polyunsaturated	
margarine	34	margarine	2
Groundnut oil	31	Soya beans	1.5
Walnuts	29	Rabbit	1
Pine nuts	25	Pine nuts	1
Sesame seeds	25	Corn oil	1
Brazil nuts	23	Groundnut oil	1
Rapeseed oil	20	Olive oil	0.5
Pumpkin seeds	20	Grapeseed oil	0.5
Linseed oil	15	Safflower oil,	
Soya beans	10.5	sesame oil,	
Almonds	10	sunflower oil,	
Cashew nuts	8	Brazil nuts, almonds,	
Olive oil	7.5	cashews, hazelnuts	trace
Linseeds	6		
Hazelnuts	4		
Quail, rabbit	trace		

† Rounded up or down to the nearest 0.5g, and is average only – content may vary according to year, season, storage times, etc.
* Alpha-linolenic acid content (EPA and DHA content of fish appears in separate chart)
** May contain less depending upon source – northern European seeds are higher in omega-3s than those from warmer climates

The main lines on polyunsaturated fat consumption

Ω Avoid sunflower, safflower and corn oil, and spreads made from these oils.

Ω Use more rapeseed oil and linseed oil (plus olive oil – see below).

Ω Eat fish, especially oily fish, regularly.

Ω Plenty of green vegetables will also help increase your intake of omega-3s (see next chapter).

Ω Do as little cooking as possible with polyunsaturated fats.

Ω Get plenty of vitamin E into your diet to help counteract the effects of oxidisation and buy, store and use your polyunsaturated fats correctly (see pages 34–5).

Mono-unsaturated fats: the unsung heroes

The last family of fats are the mono-unsaturated fats, which for years were thought to be not 'bad' for you at all – but without any particular merits, either. We now know differently about this, too.

FACT: the optimum diet for health is now thought to be one that contains adequate mono-unsaturates.

Mono-unsaturates appear in high quantities in a relatively few number of foods – olive oil, rapeseed oil, some nuts such as macadamias, hazelnuts, almonds and Brazils, and avocados. Mono-unsaturated fat also occurs in many other foods, including other nuts, seeds, meats, pulses and vegetables.

Official health guidelines suggest that around 10% of our total calorie intake should be mono-unsaturates. In the Omega Diet you will be eating more than that – around 15%, an amount that doesn't fall out of line with the official guidelines. You will be using mono-unsaturated fat to replace some of the calories you will lose by cutting right back on trans fats, saturated fats and omega-6 polyunsaturated fats. You will be using oils high in mono-unsaturated fat as your main cooking oils.

The health benefits of mono-unsaturated fats are:

Ω They lower 'bad' LDL cholesterol while keeping 'good' HDL cholesterol high, thus helping to reduce the risk of atherosclerosis, stroke and heart disease.

Ω They offer protection against some cancers. Recent research using animals has shown that olive oil offers almost the same level of protection against colon cancer as omega-3s. There is also quite good evidence to show that a diet rich in olive oil can help protect against breast cancer. And human lifestyle studies show that people living in the hot regions of the Mediterranean, who have a diet extremely high in olive oil, suffer from lower incidence of cancers, especially colon cancer, than people living in countries where high omega-6 oils are consumed for preference.

Ω They are safer to use for cooking because they don't oxidise like the polyunsaturated fats do, and are therefore much better for using at high temperatures.

Ω Mono-unsaturated fats are often high in vitamin E, the anti-oxidant which is in shortfall in many Western diets.

The most commonly used source of mono-unsaturated fat in our diet is olive oil – and much research has been done recently on this particular oil. The findings indicate that if it is good quality, extra virgin olive oil, which will contain much of the original micro-nutrients and phyto-chemicals of the olive, extra benefits accrue.

Olive oil appears to have healing and anti-inflammatory properties. It can aid digestion and enhance the work of the liver and pancreas. It contains phenols which are strongly anti-oxidant and may protect against colon and other cancers.

Mono-unsaturated fatty acid content of foods

(in g per 100g)

Olive oil	73
Shelled macadamia nuts	61
Rapeseed oil	59
Shelled hazelnuts	50
Shelled almonds	35
Shelled Brazil nuts	26
Avocado	12

The main lines on mono-unsaturated fats

Ω Oils high in mono-unsaturates are the prime oils for using in cooking. Olive oil is the best as it has the highest oxidation threshold of all the oils.

Ω Mono-unsaturated oils are an excellent all-round oil to use for general good health – high consumption has no adverse side effects, as is the case with saturates, trans fats and omega-6s.

Ω Rapeseed oil is a good oil to use because it is high in mono-unsaturates, but is also a good source of omega-3 fats. It is best used in dressings and cold dishes as it is more prone than olive oil to oxidisation.

Ω Buy your olive oil as pure and unadulterated as you can. Experiment with brands, countries of origin and flavours, as they vary tremendously.

Ω Fresh nuts are a useful source of unadulterated mono-unsaturated fats.

Introducing the four Omega Units for healthy fat consumption

Now it is time to introduce you to the first four Omega Units, which will form about a third of your daily diet and will provide most of your daily fat intake with the different types of fat in optimum balance, as well as providing many other important nutrients in your diet.

Omega Unit One

Protein Unit

Protein is one of the three essential 'macro' (meaning major) nutrients in the human diet. The others are carbohydrate and fat. So you may find it odd to have your Protein Unit in the Omega Diet described within a chapter about fats. However, almost all rich sources of protein are also sources of fat. And one of the best sources of protein – fish – is also one of the best sources of healthy fats.

As we have seen, fish, particularly oily fish, is the only real dietary source of EPA and DHA, two very beneficial omega-3 fatty acids.

Throughout the Omega Diet I would like you to consume fish at least three times a week and preferably more, and of those servings, I would like at least two and preferably more to be oily fish with the highest EPA and DHA content that you can manage.

EPA and DHA content* of selected fish

(in g per 100g)

Mackerel	2.3
Canned anchovies	2.0
Fresh herring	1.6
Canned sardines	1.6
Fresh salmon	1.4
Fresh tuna	1.2
Rollmop/canned herring	1.2
Fresh sardines	1.0
Rainbow trout	1.0
Halibut	0.9
Shark	0.8
Seabass	0.7

* Approximate only – will vary according to season, where fish is caught, cooking method and time, and other factors.

On other days your daily Protein Unit can consist of other types of protein, such as lean red meat, poultry, game, or Quorn. (See box below.) But on any day that you choose a non-oily fish item as your Protein Unit, you MUST have one to two omega-3 fish oil capsules with your meal. A source of non-polluted fish oil capsules appears in Appendix 4.

There's no need to give up meat!

Red meat is a good source of iron and B vitamins, both of which are vital in the metabolism of the essential fatty acids. You don't have to give up red meat or any other kind of meat, but on the Omega Diet there are certain points to bear in mind when choosing meat:

Ω It should be lean. Meat contains all three types of fat – and the fattier the cut, the more calories and saturated fat you are eating. So it is wise to choose lean cuts and remove excess fat, such as skin on chicken and the fat inside the bird, too.

Ω It should be free range or organic. Modern meats are higher in saturated fat than they should be because of the way the animals are farmed – using commercial feed. If an animal is allowed to graze on real grass or forage for its food naturally it will have a higher content of essential fatty acids. This is why game is good meat, and it is also why lamb has a higher EFA content than beef – even today, most sheep are kept as grazing animals, not intensively reared on bagged feed.

A guide to your Protein Unit

ONE PROTEIN UNIT equals any one of the following.

Ω *Oily fish* Small to medium portion (about 150g) oily fish from box on page 31, sardines (fresh or canned), trout, fresh tuna makes up one unit. Smoked salmon and trout and smoked mackerel will also contain good amounts of omega-3s but should only be eaten occasionally as the smoking process can leave carcinogens behind. Eat the fish skin if possible as this contains a high amount of the EFAs. Anchovies are also oily fish but it is hard to eat enough to get a portion. (Oily fish are also a good source of various vitamins and minerals in varying amounts, such as the vitamin E and B groups, calcium, iron and selenium.)

Ω *White fish* This can be a medium to large portion (200–250g) white fish – cod, plaice, monkfish, bass, haddock, swordfish, mullet, coley, hake, etc. – PLUS 1–2 omega-3 fish oil capsules. White fish is a good source of a variety of vitamins and minerals.

Ω *Shellfish/seafood* A medium portion (175g, shelled weight) of seafood – prawns, crab, scallops, lobster, mussels, squid, octopus, clams – PLUS 1–2 omega-3 fish oil capsules equals a unit.

Seafood is usually a good source of selenium, a powerful anti-oxidant, as well as zinc, magnesium and B vitamins, all of which are vital for the metabolism of fatty acids. (Try combining oily fish with seafoods to get this added bonus.)

Ω *Meat* This is a small portion (about 125g) lean fresh meat, preferably organic or free range – lean beef, leg or neck of lamb, pork fillet – PLUS 1–2 omega-3 fish oil capsules.

Ω *Poultry or game* Small to medium portion (guide – about 150g boned weight) lean poultry or game (skin removed). Free range chicken, turkey, pheasant, wild duck, pigeon, grouse, venison, crocodile, ostrich, wild boar – PLUS 1–2 omega-3 fish oil capsules is a unit.

Ω *Quorn* A medium portion (about 150g) Quorn, which is a manu-factured low-fat protein source widely available in supermarkets in the chilled counter near the meats, PLUS 1–2 omega-3 fish oil capsules is one unit. Quorn is a good source of fibre, zinc and vitamin B1.

Omega Unit Two

Oil Unit

As we have seen above, we all need reasonable amounts of fats in our diet, and the Oil Unit will provide a significant amount of this fat within your Omega Diet.

As we've also seen, the balance of fat that you eat is vital to both health and slimness – and your Oil Unit will help you to balance out your fat intake so that you get less of the omega-6s than you have probably been used to, and more of the healthy omega-3s and mono-unsaturates. (The chart on page 27 lists the omega-3 and omega-6 content of popular oils.)

ONE OIL UNIT consists of up to two level tablespoons of oil. On the 14-day diet you will often be splitting this unit into two. Sometimes you will use up to half the oil for cooking and the other half for salads. The preferred oil for the diet *when cooking* is:

* *plain olive oil* when cooking at a high temperature (as in a stir-fry, for instance); OR
* *cooking oil blend* – olive oil blended with rapeseed oil for all other cooking. To make up this blend, add 75ml of rapeseed oil for every 100ml olive oil that you use. Blend this amount and keep it in an airtight container in the fridge.

For a *salad oil blend,* mix a third each of rapeseed oil, walnut oil and groundnut oil. Make up 100ml and keep in an opaque, airtight container in the fridge. Use it up within one month.

This is a good oil for use in salads, drizzled over foods such as vegetables after cooking or stirred into soups, pasta, etc. Don't use it for stir-frying or other high-temperature cooking.

Later in the diet you can take your pick from a wider range of oils and blends, as explained in Chapter 8.

IMPORTANT NOTE ON OILS

Buy extra virgin olive oil, which has not been through a lengthy manu-facturing process which will have stripped it of much of its 'goodness'.

Buy the best quality oils you can afford, which means those that have gone through the least amount of manufacturing – heating, bleaching, etc. With oils you get what you pay for, so avoid the cheaper brands and read the label for clues as to how much processing has gone on. Natural, minimally refined oils will taste of the original food that the oil comes from: walnut oil, for instance, should taste of walnuts. These oils will contain more micro-nutrients such as lecithin (important for the metabolism of fats), vitamin E and carotene, and will be higher in the essential fats.

All oils high in omega-3s should be bought from a shop which keeps its oils in cool and dark conditions and which has a high turnover so that you can be assured that your oil is fresh and not oxidised.

At home, both the separate oils (apart from olive oil) and the oil blend need to be stored in the fridge and used up within a few weeks.

Eat as much of your Oil Unit as you can raw or very lightly heated.

Omega Unit Three

Nut Unit

Nuts are often thought of as a protein food but in fact they contain high amounts of oils which tend to be mostly mono-unsaturated plus some omega-6 polyunsaturates and very little omega-3s. Only one nut – the walnut – has good amounts of omega-3s.

The *US Nurses Study* found that frequent nut consumption in women resulted in a reduced risk of heart disease, and other studies show that regular eating of walnuts or almonds reduces LDL cholesterol in the blood.

If you buy your nuts fresh and don't store them too long, they are good unadulterated sources of the EFAs; you can eat them with confidence. If possible, buy them with shells on and only shell them when you want to eat them – they will retain more EFAs and vitamins that way and be less inclined to oxidise.

Nuts and their fat content
(in g per 100g shelled weight)

	mono-unsaturated	omega-6	omega-3
Macadamia	61	7	trace
Hazelnuts	50.5	4	trace
Pecans	45	14	trace
Almonds	35	10	trace
Cashews	28	8	trace
Brazils	26	23	trace
Walnuts	17	29	5.5

ONE NUT UNIT consists of:

A nut mix, which is a blend of 50% walnuts, 25% cashews and 25% hazelnuts. Make this mix up about 200g at a time (100g walnuts, 50g each of the other two) and store in an airtight container in the fridge.

Use this blend whenever nut mix is mentioned in the diet unless stated otherwise. An average handful of nut mix weighs around 20g, which is an average portion. This particular blend of nuts will provide you not only with a reasonable balance of oils – and a good, fresh source of unadulterated omega-6s – but also vital minerals and vitamins.

Walnuts are a good source of B vitamins, the anti-oxidant vitamin E and the mineral magnesium, a lack of which is associated with heart problems and nervous disorders. Cashews are a good source of B vitamins including folate for a healthy heart, and a wide range of minerals including the anti-oxidant selenium, iron, zinc and magnesium. Hazelnuts provide a wide range of vitamins and minerals, including vitamin E and magnesium.

Sometimes other nuts are used within the 14-day diet – say, within a recipe, or recommended within a meal. Obviously then you use the stated nuts, rather than the mix. Later in the diet, as explained in Chapter 8, you can take your pick from a wider range of nuts.

NOTE: Because of their high oil content, nuts can oxidise, just as oil does. So everything that I said above about buying and storing oils applies to fresh nuts as well, particularly those with the higher omega oil content. Buy from a good source, store them in the fridge in an airtight container and eat up within weeks. If nuts taste 'off' – bitter or rancid – then they will do you harm rather than good. Throw them away. Luckily, many nuts are good sources of vitamin E, which is an anti-oxidant.

If you cook with nuts, only lightly cook them as high temperatures and toasting/browning will accelerate the oxidisation process.

By the way, don't buy roasted and/or salted nuts (peanuts, cashews, etc.) and count them as your Nut Unit. Not only are these nuts high in salt, which we are trying to cut down on, but they have also been heated and most, if not all, of the essential fats will have been destroyed. You need fresh nuts – either in their shells or as good-quality shelled nuts. DO check the 'sell by' or 'best before' date when buying nuts.

NUT ALLERGIES: Although for most people, nuts are a good, healthy and nutritious food, quite a few of us are allergic to nuts. The most common nut allergen is peanuts, but people can be allergic to other nuts. If you have a nut allergy you will by now certainly know about it and you must avoid nuts at all costs. You should replace the Nut Unit with an extra half an Oil Unit.

Omega Unit Four

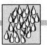

Seed Unit

Birds and many wild animals know the nutritional value of not only nuts but also seeds. In winter it is a supply of oil-rich seeds which keeps wildlife in good condition and healthy.

Humans can get the same benefits too, though the nearest most of us come to eating seeds is a sunflower seed or two in our breakfast muesli or a few poppy seeds on our bakery loaf.

Most seeds are a good source of omega-6 polyunsaturated fats and mono-unsaturated fats. The most valuable seeds from the Omega point of view are those that also contain omega-3s. Only three types of seed fulfil this criterion. Linseeds contain nearly two and a half times as much omega-3 as omega-6 fat, and pumpkin seeds contain around a third the amount of omega-3 to omega-6. Pine nuts have small amounts of omega-3 too.

Because of their extremely high omega-3 content, adding linseeds to your diet is a very easy way to alter your omega-6/omega-3 balance. Linseeds are interesting in other ways too. They are rich in lecithin, the emulsifying substance that helps in the digestion and metabolism of fats, and, according to Udo Erasmus, they increase the metabolic rate and will thus help to burn off calories. They are also an extremely rich source of lignans, a phyto-oestrogenic compound which some research has shown to fight hormone-related cancers such as breast cancer and may help to minimise menopausal symptoms.

Other health benefits Erasmus cites for linseeds are that they are anti-inflammatory, anti-bacterial, anti-fungal, anti-viral, decrease insulin resistance in diabetics, help many skin conditions, ease sore muscles and help avoid fluid retention, indigestion and constipation. If even some of these claims are correct, linseeds are powerful little seeds indeed.

Because they *are* very small, they are nearly impossible to eat on their own as a 'hand snack' – so sprinkle them on yogurt, fruit, etc., at breakfast or as part of a salad, or on top of soup or cooked brown rice.

Linseeds form part of the unit four seed mix. Pumpkin seeds are also included, not only because of their contribution to the omega-3 balance, but because they are a terrific source of zinc (for reproductive and sexual health), magnesium and iron.

The third element of the seed mix is sunflower seeds – high in natural-source, unadulterated omega-6s and mono-unsaturates, as well as vitamin E, magnesium and iron. I've included them because they are so tasty and give the seed mix an excellent touch of more-ishness. If you like, you could use pine nuts instead of sunflower seeds. They contain phytochemicals called stanol esters, which help lower cholesterol, as well as a wide range of minerals, and so are a useful addition to your seed intake.

The fat content of seeds (in g per 100g)

	mono-unsaturated	omega-6	omega-3
Linseeds	6.5	6	14
Pine nuts	13.6	25	1
Pumpkin seeds	16	20	7
Sunflower seeds	11	30.5	trace
Sesame seeds	20.5	25	trace

Most seeds contain the anti-oxidant vitamin E, which must be nature's way of keeping the oils from oxidising when stored, for as long as possible. The whole seeds are less prone, in any case, to oxidation than seed oils.

Please do try to buy organic seeds. They are such small items and have, proportionately, such a large surface area, that non-organic seeds may provide more in the way of pesticide, herbicide residues, etc., than you would want.

On your maintenance eating programme, you will be free to include a wide range of seeds, explained in Chapter 8.

ONE SEED UNIT consists of:

Ω l heaped tablespoon seed mix, made up as follows: 50% pumpkin seeds, 25% linseeds and 25% sunflower seeds (or pine nuts if preferred). Make up 100g of your seed mix at a time (50g pumpkin, 25g linseeds, 25g sunflower), stir and store in an airtight container in the fridge and use as needed.

Ω Occasionally other seed items are mentioned within the 14-day diet instead of your seed mix, but this will be made clear.

NOTE: Some people are allergic to seeds – see the note about nut allergies on page 37.

Here's a summary of the units Chapter 2 has introduced you to:

Unit One – Protein Unit

A portion of oily fish a day OR a portion of lean fish or lean meat, poultry, game or Quorn, PLUS 1–2 1,000mg omega-3 fish oil capsules.

Supplies: heart-friendly omega-3 oils, protein, B vitamins.

Unit Two – Oil Unit

UP to two tablespoons a day of either olive oil or an olive oil/rapeseed oil blend for cooking, OR a blend of rapeseed oil, walnut oil and groundnut oil for using cold.

Supplies: mono-unsaturated and polyunsaturated fats in optimum proportions, vitamin E and phytochemicals linked to very many health benefits.

Unit Three – Nut Unit

A blend of 50% walnuts, 25% hazelnuts and 25% cashew nuts every day.

Supplies: mono-unsaturated fats and some polyunsaturates, many minerals including selenium and zinc, B and E vitamins.

Unit Four – Seed Unit

A blend of 50% pumpkin seeds with 25% linseeds and 25% sunflower seeds for a rich mix of omega-3s and omega-6s, zinc, vitamin E and iron.

Now turn to Chapter 3 for an introduction to units five to eight.

Fabulous Fruits and Vegetables

Ω

Plant foods are truly nature's bounty. The colours, textures, aromas and taste sensations of bush fruits, berries, vine fruits, tree fruits, leaves, roots and so on are not just there to please the eye and other senses, but to help us to good health. With fruits and vegetables, we win all ways.

Almost all fruits and vegetables are packed with nutrients both traditional and more recently discovered. They come heavily laden with vitamins, minerals, natural sugars, fibre, digestive enzymes and a host of minute unique chemicals and organisms called phytochemicals that can do an amazing array of things to help us live long and healthy lives.

Add to that their potential to help with a slimming diet and you can see why on the Omega Diet, four of your 12 units are devoted to fruits and vegetables, as well as forming a large part of your daily 'unlimited' list.

Fruits, vegetables and slimming

First let's look at the various ways in which fruits and vegetables can help you to lose weight.

Ω *High ratio of bulk to calories* Because all fruits and vegetables have an extremely high water content, they offer you plenty of bulk/weight to 'get your teeth into' while being low, or very low, in calories. The water helps fill you up, too.

Ω *High 'crunch' factor* Eaten raw, as a large part of your fruits and vegetables will be, they also have a high 'time taken to eat' ratio compared with the calories they contain. For example, a small 25g milk chocolate bar containing 130 calories takes an average of 1 minute to eat, while an apple containing 50 calories takes an average of 3 minutes to eat. So you get three times as much eating time for just over a third of the calories.

This is mostly because lots of fruits and raw veg, like carrot and white cabbage, have a high 'crunch' factor and take a lot of chewing. The longer you take to eat foods, the less you feel like you are on a measly diet and the more likely you are to be happy about your food intake.

Ω *High satiety factor* Many fruits and vegetables are good sources of dietary fibre, which has been proven to help you feel 'full' for longer than you would expect for the number of calories you've eaten.

Fruits particularly high in fibre are many dried fruits, mango, papaya, blackcurrants, oranges, most berry fruits and pears. Vegetables particularly high in fibre are peas, broad beans, parsnips, sprouts and dark leafy greens.

Many fruits and veg are also low on the Glycaemic Index, a chart which indicates the effects that different foods will have on your blood sugar levels. A low GI factor means that that food will 'last longer' as blood glucose and, again, help you feel satisfied for longer. A steady blood glucose level also helps you to avoid side effects of poor dieting, such as dizziness, weakness, feeling faint – and hunger pangs!

Fruits lowest on the Glycaemic Index are apples, cherries, grape-fruit, pears, plums and oranges. Vegetables lowest on the Glycaemix Index are all leafy greens, peppers, onions, mushrooms, peas, beans, cauliflower and broccoli.

There is more information on the Glycaemic Index in Chapters 4 and 5.

Ω *Contain natural sweetness* Many fruits and some vegetables contain fructose or other natural sugars. These sugars are called 'intrinsic' sugar, meaning they are part of the cellular structure of the plant. This type of sweetness is perfectly acceptable as part of a diet, whereas 'extrinsic' sugars – those added to foods in cooking, at table or in the manufacturing process – are very much less of a good thing. For slimmers, extrinsic sugar is something to avoid as sugar contains no useful nutrients at all, only calories, and it often comes in the same package as fat (such as in milk chocolate) or a whole host of unnatural additives (as in packet puddings or cakes with a long shelf life).

However, because so many of us have been used to ingesting vast quantities of sugar over a long period of time, the natural sugar in fruits can come to the rescue and help to defeat our cravings for manufactured sweet foods while satisfying our sweet tooth the healthy way.

Ω *Optimum source of nutrients* When you are hungry, it is often nutrients that your body craves rather than just calories. Fruits and vegetables offer an optimum source of a wide variety of nutrients, particularly vitamins, minerals and phytochemicals, so that your body is being nourished – without the need for vitamin supplements – while the total calorie content of your diet is reduced. In other words, it is vital to eat WELL while you eat fewer calories, as otherwise you could go short of the nutrition you need for health. Fruits and vegetables help to provide that nutrition.

Here I must say a special word about seaweed. Most of us have heard of kelp. This kind of seaweed is a particularly rich source of iodine, which may be lacking in our modern diets. Iodine is vital for the correct working of our thyroid gland, which in turn controls our metabolism, growth and development. An underactive thyroid will probably result in your feeling cold, sluggish, or slow. This may result in weight gain due both to inefficient metabolism and to taking less exercise. Kelp and other types of seaweed can help to improve thyroid activity and help energy levels and, therefore, your slimming campaign, but if you suspect an underactive thyroid you should see your doctor. Seaweeds should be thoroughly rinsed before use, as they can be very salty.

Fruits and vegetables Q and A

People ask me more questions about fruit, veg and health than any other type of food. Here are some of your most frequently asked questions. I hope you find the answers helpful.

What are phytochemicals and what fruit and vegetables are they found in?

These are tiny particles which aren't nutrients as such, but are biologically active compounds which we now know can have positive effects on our health.

Phytochemicals are what give all the different plants their individual colours, aromas and so on. They are the 'factor X' which makes the plant complete and special, over and above its quota of protein, carbohydrate, fat, water, fibres, vitamins and minerals, and, surprisingly, can make up several per cent of the total weight of the plant.

All plants contain phytochemicals to some degree, but some are richer in particularly 'healthy' phytos than others. We are discovering more and more about these plant chemicals as each month goes by. Scientists have already discovered links with the prevention of major ills such as heart disease, cancer and arthritis, and with the control of the ageing process.

What some of the most important phytochemicals do will be explained in later answers to your questions in the rest of this chapter.

Are phytochemicals the same as anti-oxidants?

Although a lot of phytochemicals ARE anti-oxidants, not all anti-oxidants are phytochemicals.

An anti-oxidant is a compound – a vitamin, mineral or phytochemical – which is present in our diet and which helps us to counteract the effects of 'free radicals' which, for various reasons, may be present in excess in our bodies.

Free radicals are by-products of our bodies' production of energy and are therefore perfectly normal. But in certain circumstances there can be too many free radicals circulating – for instance, if we smoke, drink too much alcohol, are under stress, ill, dieting, take a lot of exercise, or are coping with pollutants. And in this case, it is believed, the surplus free radicals can cause cell damage, predispose to cancer and – as we found out in the previous chapter – can cause oxidisation of polyunsaturated fats and blood cholesterol in the body, thus increasing the risk of heart disease.

The anti-oxidants 'mop up' the surplus free radicals and avoid the harmful effects. The main vitamin anti-oxidants are vitamin C, vitamin E and beta-carotene (pro-vitamin A). The main mineral anti-oxidant is selenium. Some potent anti-oxidant phytochemicals are the carotenoid group, the flavonoids, and the organosulphides. All these anti-oxidants will be cropping up in answers to further questions in this chapter.

How important are fruit and vegetables as a source of vitamin C?

Very! They are our main source of vitamin C in the diet, if you exclude artificially fortified drinks, breakfast cereals, etc. Most fruits and veg contain at least some vitamin C, though some, such as citrus fruits and black and red berries, contain much more than others. (A chart of good sources appears overleaf.)

As you've seen, vitamin C is an anti-oxidant, helping to boost the body's natural defences and build a healthy immune system and healthy tissue, skin and bones, as well as helping to heal wounds.

Vitamin C has been shown to lessen the length and severity of the common cold, and new research seems to show that high levels (500mg) of the vitamin can lower blood pressure in susceptible people.

In the EC, the recommended daily amount of vitamin C is 60mg, but most experts believe this amount is too low for optimum health, and that 200mg+ may offer better disease prevention and control. On the Omega Diet you should be getting at least 200mg a day without any need to use supplements. Taking high-dose supplements of vitamin C may not be a good idea – for example, one 1999 study linked high intakes of vitamin C supplements with an *increase* in the number of free radicals produced, while another recent study linked them with increased thickening of the neck arteries. (However, more research on this subject needs to be done.)

Vitamin C content of food is easily depleted by long storage, heat, light and cooking – which is why you need to eat your veg and fruit really fresh and look after them well at home, keeping them in cool, dark conditions and cooking minimally.

Vitamin C content of fruit and veg

(in mg per 100g)

Guava	230
Red peppers	140
Blackcurrants, stewed	130
Green peppers	120
Spring greens, cooked	77
Strawberries	77
Kale, cooked	71
Watercress, raw	62
Papaya	60
Brussels sprouts, cooked	60
Kiwi fruit	60
Red cabbage	55
Mangetout	55
Oranges	55
Clementines	55
Broccoli	45
Sweetcorn, baby, cooked	40
Nectarines	37
Mangoes	37
Grapefruit	36
Raspberries	32
Peaches	31
Cauliflower	27
Satsumas	27
Spinach, baby, raw	26
Canteloupe melon (weighed without skin)	26

What other vitamins are there in fruit and vegetables?

Quite a lot – especially those coloured dark green, orange or red – are high in beta-carotene, a 'pro-vitamin' which converts into vitamin A in the body and which also is a powerful anti-oxidant. The US National Cancer Institute recommends a daily amount of 6,000ug to help prevent cancer, and research shows that adequate intake also reduces the risk of heart disease and stroke. Beta-carotene works best within a diet which is also rich in vitamin C and E (which the Omega Diet is) and is best eaten naturally within food rather than taken as a supplement. (A chart of selected good sources appears on page 50).

Quite a few vegetables, such as asparagus, avocado, kale, spinach, squash, sweet potato, tomatoes and watercress, are useful sources of the anti-oxidant vitamin E.

Some fruits and veg have good amounts of the B-vitamins in them. Bananas are high in vitamin B6, useful for women who suffer from PMS. Mangoes, broad beans, mushrooms, parsnips and peas are a good source of nicotinic acid, which is important for energy conversion and good skin. Seaweed is just about the only vegetable source of vitamin B12 and therefore important for vegans.

Blackberries, oranges, raspberries and many veg, especially green ones, are a good source of the B vitamin folate, which is vital to help reduce the amount of the chemical homocysteine in the blood. Homocysteine is, like free radicals, another by-product of energy production in the body, and raised blood homocysteine levels are linked with an increased risk of heart disease and Alzheimer's disease, among other things.

Good sources of beta-carotene

(in ug per 100g)

Carrots	8,118
Sweet potato (orange flesh variety only)	5,130
Swiss chard	4,596
Red peppers	3,840
Spinach	3,840
Butternut or other orange-fleshed squash	3,270
Kale	3,144
Spring greens	2,628
Canteloupe melon	1,998
Mangoes	1,800
Tomato puree	1,300
Cos lettuce or other dark-leaved lettuce	910
Papaya	810
Broccoli	575
Guava	435
Apricots	405
Red plums	295

What are the main phytochemicals in fruits and vegetables?

There is a large group of phytochemicals called the *carotenoids*, of which beta-carotene, discussed in the last question, is one. It is the only substance which could be described both as 'vitamin' and phytochemical as, although it isn't a true vitamin, it converts into vitamin A in the body.

The carotenoids number about 600 different compounds found in fruits and vegetables. Like beta-carotene, they often appear in greatest amounts in brightly coloured plants – green, red, orange and vivid yellow. These can either be leaves, fruit or root vegetables.

Most of the carotenoids seem to be anti-oxidant and different ones appear to work in different areas of the body. What follows is a few of the researchers' 'favourites' to date.

Lycopene is a very potent phytochemical found in greatest quantities in tomatoes, pink grapefruit, watermelon and guavas. It is at its most potent in cooked tomatoes, e.g. tomato puree or tomato ketchup or pasta sauce. It has been shown to reduce the risk of heart attacks by up to 50% and can reduce LDL blood cholesterol levels, and may also reduce the risk of some cancers, including breast cancer.

Lutein, found in dark leafy greens, blackcurrants, red peppers, sweetcorn; *beta-cryptoxanthin*, found in mangoes, peaches, papaya, oranges, tangerines and nectarines; *phytoene*, found in squash, pumpkin; and *canthaxanthin* in mushrooms have all been found to be anti-carcinogens.

Because no one can be sure yet about the interactions of these carotenoids and exactly which parts of the body which one works on, the advice is to get a wide range of brightly coloured fruits and vegetables for 'blanket coverage'.

The *bioflavonoids* are the other major group of phytochemicals in fruits.

Most active in fruits (often citrus fruits) and sweeter vegetables, they are also anti-oxidants, and help the vitamin C in our diets to be absorbed. Handily, fruits high in vitamin C are often high in flavonoids too. Flavonoids have been shown to help prevent cancers.

Taxifolin and *rutin* are flavonoids found in citrus fruits and *ellagic acid* is found in strawberries, cherries, grapes and blackberries.

A sub-group of the flavonoids are *flavonols*, including *quercetin*, an active compound in onions, tomatoes, apples, grapes and broad beans. High quercetin intake is linked with reduced risk of CHD and is anti-histamine. It can also improve lung function, even among smokers.

Resveratrol is found in red grapes, grape juice and red wine, and helps prevent CHD, while *coumarins* in several fruits and vegetables help thin the blood and prevent clotting.

Some phytochemical enzymes in fruits can aid health – *bromelain* in pineapples can help digestion and thin the blood, while *papain*, found in papaya, is also a pain-reliever.

I've heard I shouldn't eat tropical fruits but stick to fruits native to this country. Is this true?

Fruits from tropical countries, such as the pineapple, mango, papaya and banana, have been shown, in general, to have a higher Glycaemic Index (see page 44) than fruits from the colder northern European regions. So eating them may cause more fluctuations in blood sugar levels, and some people advise that we should stick to the lower GI fruits such as apples and pears.

In practice, if you eat fruit as part of a meal, rather than on its own, it doesn't really matter if the fruit has a high GI because the ingredients of the rest of the meal, if it includes protein (such as yogurt, milk, meat, fish or pulses) and fat, will lower the overall glycaemic response of the meal. And tropical fruits, as we have seen in the previous few questions, have much to recommend them in other respects – mangoes, for instance, are high in fibre, vitamin C, beta-carotene and vitamin B6.

For anyone in normal health eating normal amounts of fruit, I would say that a wide variety of fruit from all sources is a safe bet.

Which are the lowest-calorie fruits – and should I cut bananas out when slimming?

Citrus fruits are low in calories, as are rhubarb, apples, berries, kiwi fruit and melon.

In fact, most fruit is relatively low in calories despite its sweetness. This is because most are low in starch and fat and high in water. The only fruit to contain more than a trace of starch is the banana, which, weight for weight, is slightly higher in calories than most other fruit because it has much less water content.

However, as one medium banana is only around 90 calories, provides a range of nutrients AND is quite filling, I wouldn't cut them out of your diet altogether.

The avocado is the only fruit that is high in fat but again, I wouldn't cut them out of your diet long-term because they contain good amounts of mono-unsaturated fats, vitamin E and other vitamins and minerals.

Is it true that fruit is good if you have fluid retention?

Yes – many fruits (and vegetables) are a good source of the mineral potassium, which helps to regulate fluid levels in the body. It works with sodium. A high-sodium, low-potassium diet will maximise fluid retention, while a low-sodium, high-potassium one will minimise fluid retention.

A high sodium diet is to be avoided anyway as it is linked with high blood pressure and heart disease. The Omega Diet is naturally low in salt and high in potassium.

High-potassium fruits to include in your diet if you are particularly prone to fluid retention are apples, bananas, kiwi fruit, melon, papaya, nectarines, pears, plums and rhubarb. Nearly all vegetables are also high in potassium. Some of the highest are dark green leaves, onion, parsnips, cauliflower, courgettes, peas, beetroot, broccoli and cooked tomatoes.

And is it true that fruits and vegetables are high in a special kind of fibre that I won't get from cereals?

There are two sorts of fibre in the diet – insoluble fibre and soluble fibre. Grains, such as wheat, corn and rice, tend to contain most insoluble fibre, which is the sort that mostly helps you avoid constipation and helps you to feel full. Soluble fibre comes in different guises, such as *pectin, beta-glucans* and *arabinose.* These soluble fibres help to reduce LDL blood cholesterol levels and also help you maintain even blood sugar levels by slowing food absorption. Many fruits are a good source of soluble fibre (as well as insoluble fibre) and these fruits also tend to be lower on the Glycaemic Index because of the reduced rate of absorption of the sugars they contain.

Fruits highest in soluble fibre are mangoes, papaya, dried apricots, dried figs, blackcurrants, pears, prunes and oranges.

*I've read both good and bad things about dried fruits –
can I eat them or not?*

Some dried fruits are a lot better than others. All have a high sugar content (because much of the original water in the fruit has been removed and therefore they are a much more concentrated source of the sugar that was there in the first place) and therefore quite a high calorie content, but most still have a lot to offer, even for the slimmer.

Dried apricots, prunes, figs, raisins and sultanas are good sources of iron, and most dried fruits are fairly to very high in fibre (including soluble fibre, as we've just seen). Because of this, they tend to be very satisfying and filling even when eaten in small quantities.

Dried fruits feature quite often in the Omega Diet for this reason. However, I would always buy organic dried fruit, as otherwise you may end up with a diet also high in sulphates, used as preservatives in ready-to-eat dried fruits (which are partially dried and therefore keep less well than the old-fashioned well-dried kind), and in pesticides and herbicides.

*We're always told to 'eat more green vegetables'.
What are the main reasons for this?*

Several! Many dark green vegetables – such as spinach, kale, seaweed, spring greens, dark salad leaves and broccoli – are good sources of iron. They are also rich in beta-carotene and other carotenoids, which we've already discussed.

Dark green vegetables also contain essential fatty acids, a large proportion of which is the omega-3 alpha-linolenic acid – of which, as explained in Chapter 2, we should eat more. As green vegetables are a low-calorie, low-fat food, though, obviously the amount of fatty acids they contain is small. Seaweed, spinach and kale contain most – up to 2g per 100g of food – and eaten regularly, these would make a significant contribution to your fatty acid intake.

Lots of vegetables – including paler green ones and other colours, like cauliflower – are often good sources of vitamin C, calcium (which may be in short supply if you are cutting back on dairy produce – see Chapter 5) and folate.

And, just like fruit, they contain different phytochemicals which can help protect your health, and most appear to be strongly anti-carcinogenic.

Glucosinolates are a group of phytos found in broccoli, kale, sprouts, cabbage and cauliflower. They break down into other compounds called *sulphoraphanes*, which stimulate the immune system and help protect against cancer. One particular glucosinolate in sprouts, called *sinigrin*, helps to prevent cancer by killing off pre-cancerous cells in the body. And *isothiocyanate*, found in watercress, de-activates one of the main carcinogens found in cigarette smoke.

Is it true that onions are particularly good for you?

Yes, they are. Onions, along with the other members of their family – leeks, shallots, chives and garlic – are potent in *organosulphides*, another group of phytochemicals that stimulate the immune system and are anti-oxidant, a potent combination in the fight against cancer and heart disease. They help to prevent the blood from clotting, and can stave off high blood pressure, lower LDL blood cholesterol and raise HDL cholesterol. They also seem to be natural antibiotics, helping to fight bronchitis and other infections.

The onion family are also rich in potassium, fibre and vitamin C.

Get the onion family in your diet as often as you can! On the Omega Diet, they are unlimited.

Should I eat my vegetables and fruits raw or cooked?

It is a good idea to get plenty of both raw and cooked into your diet. There are advantages to each.

Raw vegetables and fruits are likely to be higher in vitamin C and B than cooked ones, as heat destroys these vitamins. As they are water-soluble, cook them without water or with very little water, to retain most vitamins. Or cook them within a casserole or compote, so that you don't throw the cooking water, and the vitamins, away.

Raw vegetables and fruits are also handy when you are slimming as they tend to take more chewing and therefore take longer to eat. Think of a raw apple compared with a couple of spoonfuls of stewed apple, for instance!

However, some vegetables and fruits can be quite indigestible to some people if they are eaten raw, and may cause either heartburn or flatulence, or both. It is much better to get your fruits and veg cooked than not at all.

And there are exceptions to the 'raw is best' philosophy.

It is known that the work of the phytochemical lycopene is more potent in cooked tomatoes than in raw ones. It is also thought that the same applies to carrots.

And, of course, some vegetables are virtually impossible to eat raw. Raw butternut squash? Raw parsnip? Raw kale? Raw artichoke? I think not.

What salads are best for me?

You'll be eating plenty of salad on the Omega Diet, as it is one good way to get your daily dose of 'raw'. Many salad items are completely un-limited on the diet so you can add them to whatever meals you like, or eat them between meals.

But when I say 'salad', what I don't mean is two small wilted leaves of lettuce, two slices of cucumber, a sprinkling of box cress and a quarter of an unripe tomato. This is an insult to salad!

What you want to do is get a nice, huge, mixed salad full of very fresh ingredients, and vary them according to what is available and in season, what costs least, what looks best, what is freshest, and what you are eating for the rest of the day.

A salad can be anything you want, from a side dish to a starter to a main course or a dessert. A good mixed salad, as a general guide, will contain a variety of dark leaves (e.g. cos, rocket, watercress, spinach, little gem), some good ripe tomato, some raw onion (red or spring is fine), at the least. But as I say, it all depends what else you're eating on the day and at the same meal. If you want a salad to go with a main course which contains red peppers and tomatoes, then you won't put red peppers and tomatoes in your salad, but stick with a variety of green things.

Use your common sense. Remember the magic word 'variety'. And do try to buy organic. If you don't buy organic, the more salad you eat the more pesticides, herbicides and so on you will also be eating.

And what about herbs and spices?

It now seems that nearly every herb and spice you can think of has some health benefit or other. Let's run through a few:

Ω *Garlic* As mentioned above, this is a member of the onion family and has the same beneficial powers as its near relations. Garlic also contains allicin, a phytochemical that has both antibiotic, anti-fungal and antiviral properties.

Ω *Chillies* These contain capsaicin, an anti-oxidant, anti-inflammatory and pain reliever.

Ω *Ginger* This stimulates circulation, and is anti-nausea and a digestive.

Ω *Coriander* A herb which is both anti-bacterial and a digestive.

Ω *Thyme* An anti-bacterial, thyme can help prevent food poisoning and chest infections, and is an anti-fungal.

Ω *Oregano, cinnamon, cloves* These three have a similar action to thyme.

Ω *Rosemary* A strong herb, this stimulates the circulation and helps minimise the length of colds and flu.

Ω *Sage* This is antiseptic, a liver tonic and a digestive.

Ω *Mint* Known as a digestive, mint is also a pain reliever.

Herbs and spices are unlimited on the Omega Diet, and full use is made of them in the 14-day diet and recipes. Now you can see why!

Here is a good place also to point out the positive properties of tea. Green tea is a powerful anti-oxidant and is a good replacement for ordinary black tea if you want a calorie-free drink without milk or sugar. However, black tea is also an anti-oxidant and a few cups a day will probably do you more good than harm.

The main lines on fruit and vegetables

Ω Get a wide variety of fruits and vegetables into your diet for the full range of benefits.

Ω Ensure you eat fruit and veg in plenty of different colours – green, red, orange, yellow, purple and white.

Ω Eat some vegetables raw at least some of the time.

Introducing the four fruit and vegetable Omega Units

On the Omega Diet, units five to eight are fruits and vegetables. They are as follows:

Omega Unit Five

C-Fruit Unit

Your C-FRUIT UNIT consists of one portion a day of a fruit or fruits rich in vitamin C. Choose from: guava, blackcurrants, strawberries, papaya, kiwi fruit, oranges, clementines, nectarines, mango, grapefruit, raspberries or a mixture of any of those.

One portion is one single large fruit (such as an orange), two smaller fruits (such as two clementines) or a good bowlful of berry fruits.

Eat your C-fruit raw.

Omega Unit Six

Fruit-2 Unit

Your FRUIT-2 UNIT consists of one portion of any other fresh fruit not included on the C-Fruit Unit list.

Your *preferred* choices are: apples, peaches, melon, cherries, red grapes, plums, pears. Each of these have their own particular special benefits, as discussed earlier in the chapter. Most are high in soluble fibre and/or low on the Glycaemic Index; others are high in a variety of phytochemicals with various health benefits.

Other fruits, such as pineapples and bananas, can be eaten from time to time as your Fruit-2 Unit, but try to choose the preferred ones as often as you can. Again, these should most often be raw, but cooked apples, plums and pears are fine now and then.

Dried fruits – certain dried fruits are also allowed. These are: dried apricots, dried figs and prunes as your preferred choices, and raisins and sultanas as second choices. These dried fruits supply fibre and iron.

A portion of dried fruit is 5 to 8 small pieces (e.g. apricot halves or prunes) or 3 to 5 larger pieces (such as figs), or a good handful of very small pieces, such as raisins.

Omega Unit Seven

Green Unit

Your GREEN UNIT consists of a large portion of any fresh mid- to dark green vegetable. Preferred choices are: kale, spring greens, savoy-type cabbage, sprouts, spinach, broccoli (calabrese) and purple sprouting broccoli. Other choices are: green beans, lettuce, broad beans, mangetout and peas. If you can get it, you can also have seaweed, such as laver or kelp. Or you can have cauliflower – although this isn't green but cream, it still contains similar phytochemicals to the others, and is also a good source of vitamin C, folate and fibre.

You can mix any of these. A large portion means a total weight of around 150g minimum – which covers about a third of an average dinner plate! Have more if you can. Any of the preferred leafy greens listed above are unlimited on the Omega Diet.

Omega Unit Eight

Flame Unit

Your FLAME UNIT consists of one medium to large portion (about 150g) of any fresh red, orange or yellow vegetable (or fruit classed as a vegetable). Preferred choices are: red peppers, yellow peppers, orange peppers, tomatoes and carrots. Orange-fleshed squash (such as butternut, Crown Prince or Turk's Turban), sweetcorn (including corn on the cob) and swede are also acceptable.

These can be eaten cooked or raw. Tomato sauce counts, for instance. The phytochemicals in cooked peppers, tomatoes and carrots may be better absorbed than those in the raw versions, but cooking destroys some of the vitamin C content – so vary between cooked and raw.

Here's a summary of the units Chapter 3 has introduced you to:

Unit Five – C-Fruit Unit

A portion of fruit rich in vitamin C.

Unit Six – Fruit-2 Unit

A portion of any other fruit including dried fruit.

Unit Seven – Green Unit

A large portion of leafy green vegetable or other preferred green vegetable.

Unit Eight – Flame Unit

A portion of red-, orange- or yellow-fleshed vegetable.

Now turn to Chapter 4 and discover an unsung nutritional hero . . .

Power-Packed Pulses

Ω

What costs next to nothing, has an almost-perfect nutritional profile and yet is just about the most neglected food group of all? It's pulses – beans, peas and lentils.

If you want good health, health protection and a great slimming tool, it's time to get wise to this fabulous family.

If your experience of eating pulses is the occasional can of baked beans in tomato sauce or a plate of chilli with red kidney beans, your heart may sink at the thought of a Pulse Unit in the Omega Diet. I think this is a great shame. The pulse family contains a rich variety of beans, peas and lentils, in all shapes, colours, textures, flavours and uses.

Boring they certainly are not. Underused, undervalued – and vastly underestimated, healthwise – is much closer to the truth.

First, let's take a look at pulses and what they can do for you. Later, I hope to convert you to their cause as a source of eating pleasure with some cooking suggestions.

The perfect profile of the pulse

If you want to eat healthily and so do your body as many favours as possible, what do you want in a food? You want one that is low in saturated fat but contains a small amount of the essential omega-6 and omega-3 fats in good ratio, that is high in soluble and insoluble fibre and full of vitamins and minerals, with a good balance of protein and carbohydrate, a low Glycaemic Index profile and preferably a 'factor X' that gives it something extra, too.

Well, in the humble bean, you have it. NO other food has all that rolled into one, so it is, without doubt, unique. Although individual varieties of bean, pea and lentil have slightly different nutritional profiles, as a family they are out there in the top league of superfoods.

Let's look a little more closely at the nutritional characteristics of the pulse.

Ω *Low in saturated fat* The total fat content of pulses varies from very low (for example, red kidney beans have less than 1g of fat per 100g) to low (chickpeas, for instance, have nearly 3g of fat per 100g). Of this fat, only between 10% and 25% is saturated. So all pulses are an extremely low saturated fat food.

Ω *Containing essential fats* The rest of the fat is mostly poly-unsaturated, and pulses are one of the few natural foods to contain reasonable amounts of the omega-3 fatty acid alpha-linolenic acid, which we looked at in detail in Chapter 2. For instance, 100g of lima (butter) beans contains 0.2g of omega-3s to 0.5g of omega-6s, giving a ratio of 5:2, and lentils contain 0.16g of omega-3s to 0.4g of omega-6s, giving a ratio of 2.5:1. The amounts of fat – with the exception of soya (see below) – are quite small, but still make a useful contribution to the day's essential fat intake.

Ω *Containing high amounts of fibre* Most pulses are good sources of both soluble and insoluble fibre, which we have already discussed in Chapter 3. Some are much higher than others. For instance, in an average 50g (dry weight) portion, dried broad beans contain 16g total fibre – nearly a whole day's adequate intake! Of that, 3g is soluble fibre which helps to keep your blood LDL cholesterol levels down and stabilises blood sugar levels. Red kidney beans contain 8g total fibre and 3.5g soluble fibre, and haricot and soya beans contain about the same. Green lentils contain 4.4g fibre, of which 1g is soluble.

So if you want a healthy cardiovascular system AND a smoothly working digestive system, then beans are your thing.

Ω *Full of vitamins and minerals* Many of the pulses are a good source of vitamin E, the anti-oxidant, so there's another plus for your heart and health. They are also a good source of several of the B vitamins, including folate, yet *another* plus for the heart (see homocysteine, page 49). And they are packed full of a variety of minerals, several of which are not all that easy to come by in the average diet. These include zinc (for its anti-oxidant and immune-strengthening properties), iron (for healthy blood and good healing potential) and magnesium (also linked with a healthy heart, strong bones and many other health benefits).

Ω *Good balance of protein and carbohydrate* Pulses are one of the few natural foods that come containing both protein and carbohydrate in almost ideal balance. About 20 to 30% of the calorie content of most pulses is protein, while about 50% of many varieties is carbohydrate. For vegetarians in particular, the protein in pulses is an important part of a healthy diet, and on the Omega Diet, where we are cutting down our animal and dairy product intake, it is just as important.

In the 'old' nutritional days, it used to be said that vegetable protein was 'second class', while animal and dairy protein was 'first class' (because the eight essential amino acids, or building blocks, of protein were not all present in vegetable protein foods, while they are in animal protein).

However, we now know that this isn't important if a varied diet is eaten. And we also know that one pulse in particular – soya – IS a complete protein (see overleaf).

Ω *Low Glycaemic Index profile* When eating few calories, as you will be doing if you follow the weight-loss Omega Diet, it is important, as we saw in Chapter 1, to choose a lot of foods from the lower end of the Glycaemic Index scale. These will help keep your blood sugar levels even and your hunger at bay. Pulses are a low GI food, most having an index of around 30, though soya is much lower than that, as we'll see. So pulses are a great food to eat when you are dieting.

Ω *The X factor* As we've seen, pulses help you to a healthy heart and circulation by helping to regulate blood fats. Pulses also contain phytochemicals called isoflavones which may offer protection from hormone-related cancers and may help in other areas, too. The soya bean (again!) contains a special type of isoflavone called genistein, which may help various female problems (see below), and which contains both cancer-fighting agents AND anti-blood-clotting agents . . .

The special soya bean

That word 'soya' has occurred several times in the paragraphs above. It is because the pale and insignificant-looking soya bean is turning out to be something of a wonder in the world of nutrition. Whatever other pulses have, the soya seems to have it bigger or better.

It contains more *fat* than other beans, at 18.6g per 100g, and is the only pulse to be used for commercial oil-making. Its omega-6 to omega-3 ratio, while not perfect, at about 6.5:1 is much better than that of most other vegetable oils (see page 27).

It is very high in *fibre* of both types, containing around 8g of fibre per 100g in total, of which 3.4g is soluble. Out of all the foods we eat only two other foods – haricots and red kidney beans – contain as much soluble fibre as this per 100g. Soya beans, therefore, have an important role to play in helping to reduce LDL cholesterol levels in susceptible people. The insoluble fibre is important for digestive health and helps you to avoid that plague of slimmers – constipation.

Soya beans have a larger range of *vitamins and minerals* in them – in good quantities – than most other beans, and rival red meat for their vitamin B content, including folate, which helps to control blood homocysteine levels (see page 49). They are also an excellent source of iron, again rivalling red meat, and a better source of calcium than most other pulses.

They are a *complete protein* too, meaning that they are the only plant food to contain all eight essential amino acids which are indispensable for adults. So again, they make a great meat substitute in the diet. In addition, their *Glycaemic Index* comes in at an extraordinarily low score of 18, making them one of the lowest GI foods around, and thus very clever at stabilising blood sugar levels – an ideal food for slimmers, and for diabetics and anyone with insulin resistance.

And lastly, they have an extra special *X factor*, as researchers are discovering. The beans' effect on LDL blood cholesterol is disproportionately high in relation to the amount of soluble fibre they contain, and it appears that other phytochemicals in the bean may be having an add-on effect. The compound genistein is probably the active factor. In any event, soya protein rich in isoflavones is so definitely linked to a reduction in LDL blood cholesterol and heart disease that in late 1999 the US Food and Drug Administration agreed that manufacturers of soya-rich foods could make claims about its health benefits on their food labels.

Genistein has also been shown to be anti-carcinogenous and can inhibit the growth of hormone-related cancers such as breast and prostate cancer. Other trials show a link between high soya protein intake and reduced risk of colon and lung cancer.

Soya beans are also described as 'nature's HRT' because they seem to help minimise the hot flushes and sweats of the menopause as well as keeping vaginal tissue healthy. Soya has also been shown to help maintain bone density in older women and thus may help to prevent osteoporosis.

Is there a downside to soya? In late 1999 an international soya symposium presented some data about possible negative properties of phyto-oestrogens (present in several plants other than soya). Over-high intakes may, for instance, suppress thyroid function, and soya formula is generally not recommended for infants, but not enough research has been done. With sensible, regular intakes it is hoped that the benefits can be enjoyed without any drawbacks – something that is true of most food. Even water is dangerous in large amounts!

The only practical drawback to soya is that the bean is not as user-friendly as some other pulses. The dried beans takes more soaking and pre-cooking than other beans, and I have known people swear that even after 12 hours of cooking soya beans are still too tough to eat! Because of their reputation, you may find soya beans harder to find in the shops than other pulses. However, if you do find them, you can soak them overnight, cook them at a rapid boil for 10 minutes and then simmer them for 3 hours; or, if you have a pressure cooker, they should cook in about 45 minutes. They can then be used in soups, salads or other dishes, particularly those including tomato, onion and red peppers.

Soya beans ARE widely available – and palatable – in other forms, which we discuss in the Q and A session at the end of the chapter.

A look at other pulses

Though soya beans may be the nutritional stars, all the other pulses are great, too. Here I run through a selection and discuss their benefits and uses in your diet.

Ω *Lentils* These are green, brown (including Puy) or red. Red lentils are lower in fibre and vitamins than the other types, so use them less frequently. Green and brown both have similar nutritional profiles, being a good source of vitamin B6 and folate, as well as iron for blood health, selenium (an anti-oxidant) and potassium for good body fluid balance. Of all the lentils, the Puy variety, from a region in southern France, have the superior taste.

All lentils are convenient because they need no pre-soaking and cook in as little as 30 minutes or so. For people who aren't used to pulses, lentils are probably the best starting point, and are ideal for soups, salads and as side dishes.

Ω *Split peas* Either green or yellow, these have less fibre, vitamins and minerals than most other pulses but are still worth including in your diet occasionally. Like lentils, they need no pre-soaking and will cook in 30 minutes or so.

Ω *Chickpeas* Not really a pulse at all, these are an 'underground nut' but are always classed with the pulses. A superb food, chickpeas are high in fibre, vitamin E, folate and iron, and contain good amounts of calcium. They're great in many Mediterranean dishes and go well with tomatoes and peppers.

Ω *Other beans* There are a wide variety of dried beans from all parts of the world. Some of the best known are the cream-coloured lima (butter) beans, which have a soft, smooth, creamy texture and flavour; red kidney beans, traditional in chilli dishes; haricot beans, the traditional 'baked bean' but good for all kinds of stews; borlotti beans, pretty yet robust Italian pink beans good for salads and savouries; blackeyed beans, good all-round beans; flageolet, pale green beans related to the haricot and used in French cooking; ful medames, or Egyptian brown beans, great with spices; and Italian cannellini beans, similar to haricots but softer and ideal in bean salads.

All these have a fairly similar nutritional profile, as described in the 'perfect profile of the pulse', above.

Pulses Q and A

How do I overcome the problem of indigestion and flatulence which I always get when I eat beans?

By no means everyone has this problem, and everyone I know has found that pulses eventually lose this effect when eaten regularly. If you are unfortunate enough to be a sufferer, you need to do three things: one, make sure that all your pulses are cooked for long enough so that they become more digestible (see below); two, increase the amount of pulses that you eat gradually over a period of 2 to 3 weeks so that your digestive system has time to adapt; and three, chew thoroughly and/or use your pulses puréed to break them down, again so you can digest them more easily. It really is worth making the effort to persist and get your body used to them. You can also buy anti-flatulence pills called Beano over the chemist's counter.

I've heard that some beans are poisonous. Is this really so?

There are toxins in some beans which are destroyed with proper cooking. Red kidney beans are a particularly high source of these toxins. What you need to do (with all dried beans except lentils and split peas, to be on the safe side) is:

Ω SOAK them overnight in plenty of water.
Ω Drain and then RAPIDLY BOIL them for 10 minutes in new water before simmering (see below).
    The rapid boiling will remove the toxins and the beans are safe to eat. All canned pulses will be safe to eat without boiling as they are pre-boiled.

How do I cook dried beans?

After the de-toxing process mentioned in the previous question, all you do is simmer for approximately one hour for most beans, or until tender. (Soya beans, dried broad beans, haricot beans and chickpeas may take longer than this – 2 to 3 hours or more.) The actual simmering time depends a lot upon the age of the bean: the longer ago they were picked and dried, the longer they will take to become tender.

Once they are cooked, you can use them in your recipes. Otherwise, if using pulses in a casserole, soup or stew, you can simply put them into your recipe after rapid boiling time, and let them simmer with the other ingredients until tender (though I wouldn't use this method for the pulses that need the longer simmering times).

How can I add extra flavour to my beans?

I have to say that I find most pulses have plenty of flavour already – and each one is different (see list on page 68). When used as part of a recipe, you don't really need to worry about adding flavour at the boiling and simmering stage.

If you are using the pulses in a salad or anywhere where flavour is paramount, you can salt the beans – but ONLY for the last 15 minutes of simmering time, otherwise they will become tough. You can also add herbs, celery, onion, leek or a carrot or two to the simmering water, which will impart a little extra flavour to the beans. You can use the simmering water to make vegetable stock as this will contain some of the B vitamins and goodness from the beans (or if you have used the suggested vegetables to improve flavour, the simmering water will already be stock, so you've saved yourself the bother).

My beans always turn out tough – why?

Either you are buying very old beans (or storing them too long), you aren't cooking them for long enough, or you are salting them early in the simmering process. Find a local supplier of pulses who has a high turnover. Sometimes chickpeas, red kidney beans and soya beans seem to be tough whatever you do with them, I will admit. In this case, use canned ones.

Are canned beans as good as home-cooked dried beans?

There shouldn't be much difference in nutrient content, although some pulses are canned in brine, which means they will have a high or fairly high salt content. Drain and rinse these thoroughly before using in your recipe. Check the label and try to buy pulses canned in water. If you live alone and don't need huge amounts of pulses at a time, cans may be your answer. Otherwise, you can cook your beans in bulk then bag them up and freeze them – they will keep in the freezer for up to three months.

Do sprouted beans count as pulses?

Fresh beansprouts -either home-grown or bought in cellophane packs in the supermarket – are excellent additions to fresh salads. The newly sprouted stems and the tiny first leaves contain vitamin C, while the seeds still contain their protein and goodness. BUT you need to eat them at just the right point – when you have just two tiny seed leaves showing, and the seed still looks fresh and fine. If you eat aged or wilted beansprouts you might as well not bother. Amost any seed can be sprouted – and of course, pulses are seeds. In the supermarket you are most likely to find sprouted mung beans or alfalfas, but at home you can try sprouting lentils, soya beans, sesame seeds – almost anything.

To answer the original question now – no, sprouted beans don't count as pulses! Sprouted pulses and other seeds count as a salad vegetable, as their nutrients are much diluted. Now much of their weight is water – so they are really low in calories, at about 32 calories per 100g, as opposed to, say, lentils, at 300 per 100g.

How can I get more soya into my diet?

You can use soya beans as described above, in soups, salads and casseroles. You can also use tofu, which is a food made from soya milk curd, which looks a bit like cheese. Tofu is a low-calorie, high-protein, low-carbohydrate food and a good source of calcium. It is available in supermarkets and health food shops in firm and 'silken' forms. The firm type can be sliced or cut into chunks and used in soups, casseroles, stir-fries and so on. The silken kind is good for dips, spreads, patés and desserts.

The downside to tofu is that it is very bland – but it does soak up the flavours of whatever you cook it with. If you marinate it according to the method on page 157, it really is very good, and can be simply grilled or baked.

Another form of soya is textured vegetable protein (TVP), which has long been used as a meat substitute for vegetarians, and is often sold as mince or chunks. This has been de-fatted, but contains all the other nutrients of the soya bean. Soya is added commercially to many processed foods such as vegetarian burgers, veggie sausages and so on. These may be good as occasional purchases, but beware: the soya in them may be genetically modified and there may be other undesirable ingredients, so read the labels carefully and go for organic products wherever possible.

Soya flour is another good purchase – it can be used to replace part of the flour in breads, cakes, pancakes and so on.

Then there are the soya condiments, such as miso, made from fermented soya beans and used to enrich casseroles, soups, etc. Soya sauce, by the way, contains very little soya as such and is high in salt, but is still good for occasional use as a tasty low-fat condiment.

In Chapter 5 we discuss two forms of soya that really do make life easy if you want to increase your soya intake. These are soya milk and soya yogurt, which can both replace the dairy versions in your diet.

I have high blood cholesterol. How much soya do I need to get in my diet to make a difference?

Research has showed that 25g of soya protein daily may help to reduce the risk of heart disease, and as little as 20g a day has been shown in one study to lower LDL blood cholesterol levels. This is roughly equivalent to one serving of soya beans, TVP or tofu or two glasses of soya milk.

A measure of 40g a day has been shown to significantly increase spinal bone density in postmenopausal women. And one trial showed that 39g of soya protein daily reduced the risk of precancerous colo-rectal tissue.

Not enough research has been done on the effects of other pulses to predict how much of them is needed for health protection, but a daily portion will certainly offer optimum nutrition, as described under 'The perfect profile of the pulse' on page 63.

Omega Unit Nine

Pulse Unit

Every day you'll have one PULSE UNIT, which is simply one medium portion (about 150g) of cooked beans, peas or lentils OR tofu OR textured vegetable protein.

Try to have soya beans or tofu at least 2 to 3 times a week, especially if you aren't going to use soya milk and yogurt instead of dairy milk and yogurt in your Calcium Unit (see Chapter 5).

Some examples of preferred Pulse Units are:

Ω *Peas* These can be split yellow or green peas or chickpeas.

Ω *Lentils* Choose brown or green for preference.

Ω *Beans* These include soya, red kidney, blackeyed, borlotti, black, butter (lima), cannellini, broad, flageolet, ful medames (Egyptian brown beans), haricots, pinto, baked beans in tomato sauce.

Ω *Other* Or have lentil paté, hummus (chickpea purée) or any other pulse purée

CHAPTER 5

The Big Three for Energy

Ω

This chapter introduces you to the last three Omega Units. The first, Quality Carbs, you will easily recognise as an important part of your diet. The second and third may surprise you. But all three have a vital role in your health and energy levels.

Quality carbohydrates

Carbohydrates are, in one way, a lot like fat. As we saw in Chapter 2, fats can be very, very bad or very, very good, and so can carbohydrates. And yet in the Western world it is the less good carbohydrates, just like the poor fats, that form the bulk of our starch intake.

On the Omega Diet you will be eating only what I term 'quality' carbohydrates – the starchy carbohydrate grains and roots which enhance the total nutritional quality and balance of your diet and which have positive effects on your health.

The difference you will find through eating only such carbohydrates and avoiding the poor ones will, I am sure, be immense.

What starch does for you

Carbohydrates come in two types – sugars and starches. In the main, the sugar carbs in the Omega Diet are provided by the fruit units. In the main, the starches are provided by the Quality Carb Unit. The main sources of starch in the diet are grains and root vegetables.

Starch is important in the diet as the preferred provider of energy for everything that we do. It converts readily into energy in the body, whereas fat and protein follow a more roundabout route. But grains and roots in their natural form also provide us with important nutrients – vitamins, minerals – as well as important fibre, and some fat and protein too. Most grains are particularly good sources of the

B vitamins, vital for energy metabolism and for helping us to feel full of energy ourselves.

What has gone wrong in the typical modern diet is that the starches we eat are mostly highly refined – grains have been milled, ground and altered so that there is little of the original goodness left. So little, in fact that manufacturers in the UK have for years actually added artificial vitamins and minerals to make up for what has been lost from the natural product – and on the packs seem to claim that they should somehow be praised for this! Also, most of the original fibre and the small amounts of essential fats have gone. And this is the starch that we consume in vast quantities in our factory-made white bread, our factory-made breakfast cereals, our highly refined quick-cook white rice and pasta, our cakes, our biscuits, our pastries and pies . . . Reading most of the packets on these products, you would hardly believe just how unnatural many of them are.

The World Health Organisation urges us to eat around 50% of our daily calories in the form of carbohydrate. But it means *good quality* carbohydrate, from natural sugar sources and from natural grain and vegetable sources, not processed pap.

For slimmers, refined carbohydrates spell disaster, as we fill ourselves up with junky baked goods and cereals which do little to satisfy our cravings. As we've seen, our bodies crave nutrients and good nutrition, not just calories! If you eat a plate of white bread with syrup or processed spaghetti hoops you're getting carbohydrate, sure, but little fibre, little essential fats, only synthetic vitamins in the main (and very few at that) and nothing that your body can really enjoy. Your mouth may enjoy it – but when the food gets as far as your stomach, your body won't.

And there's one more reason for this.

The Glycaemic Index

I've mentioned the Glycaemic Index before. It's the index that shows how quickly or slowly a carbohydrate food is absorbed into the bloodstream, and then dissipates. Foods that are high on the GI are very quickly absorbed. Foods that are low are slowly absorbed. And high-index foods have your blood sugar levels fluctuating, and create an overworked pancreas (which is responsible for releasing insulin to cope with the sugar in the blood and help it to be absorbed), which may then lead to what is termed insulin resistance and the various negative symptoms that come with low blood sugar/high blood sugar fluctuations. These can include hunger, weakness, dizziness, lack of concentration and perhaps, in the long term, non-insulin-dependent diabetes and obesity.

Foods that are low on the GI, however, have a positive effect on maintaining even blood sugar levels by releasing their sugars slowly into the bloodstream, and by taking longer to be absorbed and letting the pancreas and insulin do their job slowly and without any hassle. Result – much less insulin resistance, less overeating, less chance of diabetes, a properly working digestive system, no symptoms of hypoglycaemia, a happy body, and therefore a happy person.

This is why, in the main, the carbs that you will be eating on the Omega Diet are mainly low or medium on the GI, and not high. I don't always pick the lowest-GI foods because you have to balance their GI with the nutrients the foods contain and come up with a sensible compromise. For your interest, a description of natural or nearly natural carb foods, with their GI rating, appears overleaf. Over 70 is high, under 40 is low.

NOTE: Another way to slow the rate of absorption of carbs and therefore keep blood sugar levels even is to add fat or protein to your meal. Both fat and protein take longer than even low-GI carbs to be absorbed. On the Omega Diet, the fats and proteins that you add to your carbs will all be good for you. This adding of fats and proteins is more important when choosing GI carbs at the higher end of medium (such as a slice of wholewheat bread, which has a GI rating of 69) rather than the lower-rated ones (a slice of pumpernickel bread, for example, which has a rating of 41).

The different types of quality carbohydrate

Now we need to look at the different starches and weigh up their 'pros' and 'cons', picking only the best for the Omega Diet. First let's look at grains, which will form the bulk of your Quality Carb Units.

Grains are the staple foods of the world because they are easy to grow or inexpensive to buy, and can sustain life.

Ω *Wheat* This is the big one in the UK as it is our native grain. Much of the bread, baked goods and breakfast cereals that we buy are based on wheat, but sadly, most are the refined versions. Wholewheat is a good source of the B vitamins, vitamin E, iron, protein, fibre, may be a good source of selenium (see the first question in the Qs and As below) and also contains essential fatty acids. Its GI depends upon how it is prepared. For example, an ordinary slice of wholewheat bread has a GI of about 69, whereas a piece of wholewheat pitta bread has a GI of only 57 and cracked wheat (bulghar wheat) only 48. Wholewheat pasta has an even lower GI at 40, and, surprisingly, even white pasta comes in quite low at 50, although as white pasta is much lower in fibre and nutrients than wholewheat, it doesn't rate as a quality carb – at least, not in this book!

Good as wheat is, we probably overuse it, and on the Omega Diet I bring in a selection of other grains to add a wider variety of nutrients and for other more specific reasons.

Ω *Rice* This grain deserves to be much more popular than it is. I never know why people call it boring. Wholegrain (brown) rice is also a good source of B vitamins and magnesium, fibre and other trace elements. Rice is also a suitable grain for people who are gluten intolerant (see Qs and As below) and is less likely to cause stomach bloating, wind and fluid retention than is wheat.

Interestingly, both brown and white rice have a higher GI than you would imagine. Standard brown rice has a GI of 76, standard white rice a very high 87. This is because standard rice is high in amolypectin, a type of starch which breaks down quickly. However – thank goodness for basmati rice, the 'king of rices' from India. Not only does it taste the best of all the rices and cook well, it is also high in a different starch, amylose, which has the reverse effect. White basmati rice has a score of 58 and brown basmati a score of 55, so when choosing rice, always choose brown basmati if you can for all the benefits of rice and none of the drawbacks.

Ω *Rye* A much-neglected grain in the UK, rye is a good source of iron, phosphorus, calcium, vitamin E, B vitamins and fibre. It contains less gluten than wheat. Pumpernickel bread has a 41 GI value, and standard dark rye bread 65. Dark rye crispbreads are a valuable alternative to breads for people with a yeast intolerance, as they contain no yeast.

Ω *Oats* These are one of the few cereals rich in soluble fibre, and regular intake has been clearly linked with lowered LDL blood cholesterol levels. For a cereal, it has a very low GI index of 49. Oats also have a higher fat content than most cereals, with a good amount of omega-3s in them as well as omega-6s, and are rich in iron and zinc. Oats can be used not only as a breakfast cereal (in porridge or muesli) but also in bread. Traditional savoury oatcakes (flat biscuits), with a GI of 55, make a good alternative to cream crackers, with a GI of 75. Quick-cook oats (instant breakfast cereal) are much less rich in the nutrients and fibre and are best avoided.

Ω *Barley* The wholegrain 'pot barley' kind is also rich in fibre of both kinds, iron, potassium, phosphorus and the B vitamins, and is excellent in casseroles, soups and salads. It also has an extremely low GI rating of 22 and thus is worth including in any slimming diet.

Ω *Corn* Maize is a useful grain for bread, puddings and so on if you are gluten intolerant, as it contains none. It is lower in the typical grain nutrients – B vitamins, fibre, magnesium and so on – than other grains, but is a good source of iron. As a substitute for rice, pasta or potatoes, it is often served as polenta, which sadly is fairly bland and tasteless unless lots of cheese, butter and so on are added. Corn also has a relatively high GI index rating, in comparison with several other grains, at 68. As it isn't such an all-round 'good' grain as most of the others, I include it, used as a grain, hardly at all on the Omega Diet. But it can be eaten as fresh or frozen corn on the cob when it would count as a Flame vegetable.

Ω *Buckwheat* This isn't a wheat at all and contains no gluten so is good for wheat- and gluten-intolerant people. Cracked and toasted it is called kasha and is much eaten in this form in eastern European countries. It has a reasonable GI value of 54 and contains good amounts of selenium and zinc. Buckwheat flour is good used in flatbreads and pancakes. You can also buy buckwheat pasta and noodles, which are useful, again, if you are allergic to wheat.

Ω *Quinoa* A small grain growing in popularity in the UK, quinoa can be boiled and eaten like rice. It is very high in protein for a grain, rich in nutrients and likely to have a low GI rating, although it isn't on the current list of GI foods, and is worth trying for a change from the more usual grains. *Amaranth* grain is rich in iron, potassium and calcium and becoming more available, and *millet* is also another high-protein grain, also high in phosphorus, iron and potassium, which you may like to try once in a while. All three are gluten-free.

The other main source of starch in the diet is certain root vegetables, the most common of which is the *potato*. Potatoes are a reasonable source of fibre, potassium, vitamin B6 and vitamin C (although levels of these vitamins diminish when the potato is stored). They contain a small amount of protein and hardly any fat. They also benefit from being inexpensive and familiar, with a certain 'comfort food' element about them. For some reason, boiled potatoes (at 56) have a lower GI than mashed (70) or baked (85), and new potatoes contain more vitamin C than old. So the preferred potato on the Omega Diet is new, boiled potatoes. However, other forms of potato – particularly baked or whole-roast in olive oil – are perfectly fine for less frequent use.

Even better than standard potatoes are *sweet potatoes* or *yams*. Here I am talking about the kind of sweet potato with bright orange flesh. Sometimes in the shops they will be labelled as such, other times as yams. Either way, if you surreptitiously scrape a tiny bit of skin you will see whether the flesh is orange or not. If it is pale cream-coloured, it won't contain all the carotenoids which are so good for health (see page 50).

Sweet potatoes taste delicious, are high in vitamin E and C as well as potassium, and have a reasonable amount of fibre. They also contain phyto-oestrogens, which appear to be helpful to menopausal women. With a GI of only 54, sweet potatoes are worth including in your diet regularly.

Parsnips, while not included on the 14-day Omega Diet as they have an extremely high GI factor at 97, are nevertheless good carbohydrate food, too. These roots are rich in beta-carotene (even though they aren't orange), B vitamins including folate, vitamin C, potassium, phosphorus and iron. They are very high in fibre for a root veg, and contain phytochemicals called terpenes, which have been linked with the ability to discourage the spread of cancer growths. You will be able to eat parsnips on the Omega Plus maintenance plan.

Carbohydrates Q and A

Which starches are the best to eat to avoid cancer?

There is fairly strong evidence linking a high intake of cereals with lowered risk of bowel cancer and some evidence with lowered risk of pancreatic cancer. Both these lowered risks are thought to be because a high (wholegrain) cereal diet contains high levels of insoluble fibre. Wholegrains also contain lignan, the compound similar to fibre which has an oestrogenic effect and may reduce the risk of hormone-related cancers, such as breast cancer. If you eat refined cereals, of course, you won't get this benefit.

There is also evidence linking a diet high in the mineral selenium with at least a 50% reduction in the risk of men getting prostate cancer – the third biggest cancer killer in the UK. Wholewheat is – or should be – rich in selenium, and buckwheat, soya flour and oats all contain good amounts too.

A recent review by the Dunn Clinical Nutrition Centre in the UK stated that up to 80% of bowel and breast cancer may be preventable by dietary change.

Is there any link between eating starch and lowered risk of heart disease?

Several studies in the 1980s linked a high intake of oats with a lowered risk of heart disease. This is thought to be because of the high amount of soluble fibre oats contain.

Several other studies in the past few years have shown a decrease in the risk of heart disease in people who eat a diet high in wholegrains of any kind. A huge 1995 study at Harvard University in the US showed that men who ate high-fibre diets reduced their risk of CHD by one-third – and the strongest association with a reduced risk was with fibre from cereals.

In 1999, another large American study of postmenopausal women who ate a high-cereal diet found that they had a third less chance of dying of a heart attack than women who didn't.

Most cereals contain good amounts of the B vitamin folate, which has been shown to reduce levels of homocysteine in the blood (see page 49), and this could be one reason why they work to help prevent heart disease.

Do cereals have any other major health benefits?

They are generally good for your digestive system, helping to keep constipation at bay, and with their high and wide-ranging nutrient content are an important (and inexpensive) part of a healthy diet. There is evidence that a high-fibre, high-cereal diet can help to prevent diverticular disease, a common complaint in older people.

I think I am allergic to wheat and gluten – what starches can I eat?

Do you know for certain that you are allergic to wheat and gluten? If so, of course you can eat the starchy root vegetables such as potatoes, parsnips and sweet potatoes. You can also eat certain grains. Wheat and rye contain gluten, and barley and oats contain gluten-like substances which are usually also badly tolerated by people allergic to wheat and gluten, and so all these are best avoided (sadly). Some gluten-intolerance sufferers may find, however, they *can* tolerate oats. Good substitutes are buckwheat, rice, wild rice, millet, amaranth and quinoa.

Some people may be mildly allergic to wheat without a genuine gluten intolerance, finding that a high-wheat diet produces stomach bloating, fluid retention, tiredness and weight gain. If that sounds like you, try excluding wheat for a month. Rye, barley and oats may all be fine if you have this condition, but a good plan is to exclude all four for the month and then reintroduce them in this order – oats, barley, rye, wheat – a week at a time each. If your symptoms return when you introduce one of these, you know you have your culprit. If excluding wheat doesn't relieve your symptoms, the cause could be many other things and you should see your doctor for a referral to a nutritionist.

Genuine gluten intolerance, known as coeliac disease, is a serious condition and should be medically treated.

If I have a yeast allergy, what grain products can I eat?

Most raised breads include yeast, but yeast-free starches include soda bread, chapatis, ricecakes, rye crispbreads and all breads labelled 'yeast-free' (often sold at health food shops and in the specialist section of supermarket bread counters). You can also, of course, eat pasta and all the grains in their whole, cracked or rolled form – bulghar wheat, rice, oats and so on.

Is it okay to eat pasta?

Pasta made from the wholegrain of wheat (wholewheat pasta) is fine – it is a mix of flour and water (though check the label, some pastas do contain egg). Pasta also benefits from having quite a low GI score, of around 40 (depending upon the shape – thicker pastas such as papardelle have a lower GI, thinner ones such as vermicelli a higher one).

Omega Unit Ten

Quality Carb Unit

While slimming, you will be eating slightly less of the quality carbs than you will later, on your maintenance diet. You can, if you like, split your Quality Carb Unit into two each day, or else take it all in one go if you prefer. Don't forget to vary your choices of carbs as much as possible for a wide variety of nutrients.

ONE QUALITY CARB UNIT consists of one medium portion quality carbohydrate, as follows:

Ω Any wholegrain bread including wholewheat, black rye, oat, mixed grain. A medium portion is about 80g (three slices).

Ω One large wholewheat pitta or chapati.

Ω Up to four plain oatcakes.

Ω Up to six dark rye Ryvitas.

Ω Wholewheat pasta. A medium portion is about 60g (dry weight).

Ω Wholegrains – brown rice (preferably brown basmati), pot barley, oats, bulghar wheat, buckwheat, quinoa, millet, amaranth. A medium portion is about 60g (dry weight).

Ω Wholegrain breakfast cereal – shredded wheat, old-fashioned porridge, All-Bran, muesli (with no added sugar or salt), puffed wheat, Weetabix (about 50g)

Ω New potatoes in their skins. A medium portion is about 225g.

Ω Sweet potato, one whole medium.

Ω Parsnip. A medium portion is about 225g.

Ω OR 2 × half portions of any of the above.

Calcium: a king of minerals

Calcium isn't a 'trendy' mineral, like selenium, or an exciting new discovery, like phytochemicals, but it is certainly an extremely important part of a healthy diet for many reasons. And, especially for people cutting down on their saturated fat and calorie intake, it is surprisingly hard to get adequate amounts in your diet. That is why one of my 12 Omega Units is devoted to calcium.

With your Calcium Unit, you will not only be ensuring you get enough of 'the white stuff', you will also be getting 'booster doses' of other important nutrients, and one or two 'bonus extras' as well.

But first let's look at calcium itself, and what it does for you and your body.

Bone health through life

Calcium is the major mineral in your bones and teeth, making up about 1kg of the weight in the 'average' adult body. To build to these levels in childhood and young adulthood, and to maintain bone strength and density in adulthood and old age, you need a regular intake of calcium of about 1,000mg (1g) a day.

Without adequate calcium intake (and other correct nutritional factors – see the Q and A section below) children may not reach 'peak bone mass' (that is, have as good and strong a skeleton in young adulthood as would be possible with optimum intake), and adults may not maintain it. Peak bone mass is important because with age (and, in women, with the menopause), bone tends to lose its density and strength, which can lead to osteoporosis, fractures, spinal curvature and other skeletal problems. And if this happens, you lose your mobility. Basically, if you haven't got a firm structural foundation, you haven't got health, and the slimmest, prettiest appearance won't count for much either. It is VITAL to do your best to maintain your bones in good order.

Calcium for your heart

The links between calcium intake and the health of your heart and cardiovascular system are very strong. Firstly, a high calcium intake seems to reduce blood pressure. High blood pressure (hypertension) is one of the major risk factors for heart disease. Some experts believe that a high calcium intake is even more important than a low sodium (salt) intake in reducing blood pressure.

There is also circumstantial evidence linking hard water areas (where tap water contains high amounts of calcium) with reduced incidence of heart disease.

Calcium for your energy, muscles and nervous system

All your muscles (including the heart) need adequate calcium to function smoothly. Symptoms of deficiency include muscle weakness and cramps. Calcium is also needed for nervous health: it is well known that a mug of hot milk – rich in calcium – will help relax you and give you a good night's sleep. A lack of calcium can hinder your general metabolic processes and may have you feeling tired, lethargic, lacking in energy and 'off colour', while not exactly ill.

Getting calcium into your diet

Dairy produce For most people on a typical Western diet, the main source of calcium is dairy produce – cheese, milk, yogurt and ice cream. However, the cheeses highest in calcium, such as Cheddar and Gruyère, are also high in saturated fat and calories, and therefore absent from the Omega Diet. Low-fat cheeses like cottage cheese are lower in calcium as well. Ice cream is high in fat and/or sugar and usually high in calories too, so it's best avoided.

The best dairy products for getting your calcium without the fat and/or calories are skimmed milk (at 120mg per 100ml) and low-fat yogurt (at 190mg per 100ml). Low-fat fromage frais has much less calcium than yogurt, at about 90mg per 100g, but still more than cottage cheese at 73mg per 100g. Both fromage frais and cottage cheese have more calories per 100g than skimmed milk and low-fat yogurt, so the calcium to calories ratio is low. When you're watching calorie intake, the more calcium you can get for your calories, the better, so on these terms low-fat yogurt (preferably bio yogurt – see box opposite) and skimmed milk are almost identical. Just 200mg of yogurt or 300ml of milk will supply nearly half of your daily calcium needs.

Soya There is a lot to be said for swapping your daily dairy produce for an alternative soya version. Both soya milk and soya yogurt are naturally low in calcium, but they both come in calcium-enriched versions and are extremely low in calories, with a good calcium to calories ratio (see box).

The advantages of soya are many, as you will recall from Chapter 4, which discussed pulses (see pages 66–7). To recap: soya is good for the heart, helping to reduce LDL blood cholesterol. It can probably help reduce the symptoms of menopause, such as hot flushes – and, more importantly in this context, appears to also help prevent loss of bone density (first sign of osteoporosis) in postmenopausal women. In other

The benefits of bio

The other benefits of low-fat dairy produce are that they are high in protein, contain B vitamins (again for energy, and general good health, including a healthy nervous system) and, if you buy low-fat bio yogurt, contain important 'friendly' bacteria – usually acidophilus and bifidus – which can colonise the gut, help to improve the immune system and perhaps even help prevent cancers and heart disease. If you have been eating a poor diet, have been ill or taking antibiotics, your friendly gut bacteria may be depleted and in need of help. Bloating and wind, irritable bowel, thrush and tiredness are all possible signs that you may need more 'probiotics', as the bacteria are known. There are no probiotics in skimmed milk, so low-fat bio yogurt should be included as your calcium unit on a regular basis.

Calcium and calories (ml per 100g of food)

	calcium (mg)	calories	ratio
Skimmed milk	120	33	3.6:1
Low-fat bio yogurt	190	56	3.4:1
Low-fat fromage frais	90	112	0.8:1
Cottage cheese	73	98	0.7:1
Calcium-enriched soya milk	140	45	3.1:1
Calcium-enriched soya yogurt	140	72	1.9:1

words, if you take soya milk enriched with calcium, you get a double-whammy of help with your bones. Soya milk also contains good levels of protein, vitamin E and B vitamins.

Other sources The rest of your day's calcium intake will come from the other Omega Units. Green leafy vegetables, nuts and seeds, white fish and small fish such as sardines all help build your calcium profile. The Water Unit will provide you with calcium too.

Calcium Q and A

I don't like milk. Can't I just take a calcium supplement?

These aren't usually as well absorbed by the body as calcium in foods. Only about 40% of the calcium you eat is absorbed anyway, and absorption is helped by a diet rich in essential fatty acids, vitamin D (present in large amounts in oily fish) and magnesium (in nuts, seeds and wholegrains).

As we've seen, low-fat bio yogurt is an even better bet than milk, so you could use that instead. Certainly, a calcium supplement, especially when taken halfway through a meal, is better than nothing. Find one labelled calcium citrate, which, tests show, is more easily absorbed than other formulations. Have extra portions of leafy greens, nuts and seeds, too.

Is it all right to have my daily milk unit in cups of tea and coffee?

As you've seen, tea and coffee should be limited on the Omega Diet. But there is a good reason not to take your milk this way – the tannin in tea and coffee hinders the absorption of calcium.

Omega Unit 11

Calcium Unit

There isn't a very broad choice for your Calcium Unit. The preferred unit for most days is low-fat bio yogurt because, as we've seen, not only does it have a good calcium to calories ratio, but it also contains probiotics. Try to eat bio yogurt regularly. The second preferred choice is calcium-enriched soya milk, with its great nutritional profile. The third choice is ordinary skimmed milk – low in calories, high in calcium, but with none of the added benefits of soya or bio yogurt. If you like, you can use half dairy bio yogurt or milk, and half soya yogurt or milk. This way you get all the benefits.

Other sources of dairy or soya calcium can be eaten from time to time. Just taken occasionally, low-fat fromage frais, cottage cheese and soya yogurt add interest to your diet. Very occasionally, you can have half-fat Greek yogurt.

ONE CALCIUM UNIT equals:

Ω 200g low-fat bio yogurt or calcium-enriched soya yogurt.
Ω 300ml skimmed milk or calcium-enriched soya milk.
   OR 2 × half portions of any of these in any combination.
Ω 100g low-fat fromage frais – occasional use only.
Ω 100g cottage cheese – occasional use only.
Ω 100g half-fat Greek yogurt – very occasional use only.

Revive your thirst for water

Finally, let's drink to the last Omega Unit of the 12. No, sorry – it isn't wine. It's WATER. Water is the often forgotten element of a healthy diet and of a slimming diet. Here I explain why it is so important to you.

You are 75% water – at least in an ideal situation. In fact, one recent study found that up to half of us don't drink enough water to keep our bodies hydrated, which leads to all kinds of health and functioning problems.

Lack of water hinders the work of the kidneys and liver, causes digestive problems, may lower the absorption of nutrients, can affect mood and our looks – and much else. As the brain is up to 85% water, dehydration can have many effects on our mental functioning too.

But how can you tell if you are dehydrated? Here are the signs:

Ω Constipation
Ω Infrequent visits to loo
Ω Dark-coloured urine
Ω Dry skin, hair and nails
Ω Palpitations or increased pulse rate
Ω Headache
Ω Fatigue
Ω Poor concentration
Ω Dry mouth and furry tongue
Ω NO sweat even though doing hard physical exercise
Ω Thirst (but you don't have to feel thirsty to be dehydrated)

How water helps your body

Ω *Healthy digestive system* As we've seen, a high fibre intake is important to help prevent constipation and colon cancer, among other things. But fibre can't do its work unless you increase your fluid intake, too. If you are dehydrated, your body tissues hold on to all the water they can find, so there is little left for the fibre to soak up and thus increase the bulk of the stools, which is what prevents constipation. And water may also help fight colon cancer. One study found that increasing water consumption may cut a woman's risk of getting colon cancer by up to 50%.

Ω *Healthy skin, hair and nails* Water hydrates the whole body, and is nature's moisturiser for the skin. If you suffer from dry or dull skin, the first thing to do is increase the amount that you drink. No amount of creams in a jar will help if you are dehydrated. Long term, the condition of your hair and nails will also improve.

Ω *Helps keep kidneys and liver healthy* Both need plenty of water so that they can do their daily job – to filter and rid the body of waste products and toxins. Adequate water helps prevent kidney stones and reduces the risk of cystitis. Dark urine is a sure sign that you aren't drinking enough to help these organs work efficiently.

Ω *General improved well-being* Symptoms that you may consider almost normal – or may blame on something else, like a food allergy or PMS – such as headaches, irritability, lassitude and lack of concentration, may actually be caused by dehydration. Symptoms should improve within days if dehydration is the real cause.

How water helps in your slimming campaign

Ω *Reduces fluid retention* It is a myth that increasing fluid intake means increased fluid retention: the opposite is nearer the truth. If you drink a lot of water, it dilutes the levels of sodium (salt) in your body tissues and helps to flush them out. A high sodium intake is linked with fluid retention.

Fluid retention is very depressing if you are overweight, as there is always the tendency to think that it is fat, even when it isn't.

Ω *Helps blunt the appetite* Tests show that if you drink a glass of water a few minutes before a meal, you will tend to eat less. Sipping a glass during your meal will slow down the time it takes to eat and thus help you to feel satisfied at the end of the meal. (Studies show that the longer your meal takes to eat, the more the 'satiety' mechanism has time to click into place and inform you that you are full!) Lastly, if you feel peckish between meals and have a drink of water, it will help prevent you from snacking on high-calorie nibbles.

Ω *Contains no calories* Water is the only thing you can eat or drink that has absolutely no calories in at all. Therefore it is the ideal drink to use to replace higher-calorie alternatives that you've forsaken. Sparkling water with some lemon or lime juice and some ice is a tasty and refreshing alternative to wine, or any other alcoholic drink, for that matter. It is also infinitely nicer than diet fizzy drinks (see Questions and Answers, below).

Ω *Helps remove toxic by-products of dieting* When you are dieting, the liver processes the fat that has been stored in your fat cells but is now released into the bloodstream and used as fuel. This process produces toxins, which water helps remove from the system. Water also helps the metabolic system to work efficiently.

Ω *Helps you to exercise* Water helps to keep your joints and muscles mobile and prepared for exercise, and to absorb shock, and hydrates you during and after exercise, helping to prevent exhaustion.

Water Q and A

How much water should I drink a day, then?

You should aim to drink a minimum of six glasses of water a day, evenly spaced out, each glass about 8 to 10 fl oz (225ml to 300ml), making a total daily water intake of about 1.75 litres or three pints. This is a ballpark figure, as lifestyle and other factors will affect exactly how much you need. If you are very active and/or the weather is hot you will need more. If you are sedentary and it is cold you may get by on less. Body weight is another factor – heavier people need more water.

One equation that may help you work out your own needs is the American standard of $\frac{2}{3}$ fl oz water for every pound of body weight a day for an active person and $\frac{1}{2}$ fl oz for an inactive person (see chart opposite).

You will also be getting water from the food that you eat. On the Omega Diet you have a high intake of fruit and vegetables, which have a very high water content.

Incidentally, you can drink TOO much. Twelve litres a day or more can cause real health problems, including kidney strain and low sodium levels. Several litres of water drunk all at one go can even cause death! Be sensible!

Don't drinks such as cola, coffee, tea and alcohol count towards my daily fluid intake?

All four of those are diuretics, meaning that they tend to deplete the body's fluid levels rather than enhance them, so they can't be counted towards your fluid intake.

On the Omega Diet you can have other drinks in addition to your six glasses of water – all the allowed drinks are shown on the unlimited list on page 105. These include such things as herbal teas and green tea. You can also flavour your water with lemon or lime juice. Once you get used

Optimum daily fluid intake for adults

Weight	Active person		Inactive person	
	pints	litres	pints	litres
9 stone	4	2.3	3.2	1.8
9 stone 7lb	4.4	2.5	3.3	1.9
10 stone	4.6	2.6	3.5	2.0
10 stone 7lb	4.9	2.75	3.7	2.1
11 stone	5	2.9	3.8	2.2
11 stone 7lbs	5.3	3	4	2.3
12 stone	5.5	3.1	4.2	2.4
13 stone	6	3.4	4.5	2.5
14 stone	6.5	3.7	4.9	2.8
15 stone	7	4	5.3	3

to drinking more water it will become highly palatable. There is a huge variety of bottled waters, all of which have their own individual flavour. There is no harm in the occasional cup of (weakish) black tea as this, too, is an anti-oxidant. But don't count it towards overall fluid intake!

Can I drink tap water or does it have to be bottled?

Yes, you can drink tap water. All the tap water in this country is supposed to be safe to drink and contains a range of minerals such as calcium and magnesium, which have been shown to help reduce the risk of heart disease. Some studies have shown less desirable chemicals in tap water – pollutants of various kinds, such as pesticides and antibiotic residues. However, these are deemed by the government to be present in safe levels. Arguments rage almost constantly about water fluoridation and chlorination. If you are worried about your own tap water, you can ask your local water authority for an analysis of its contents and then decide if you want to play safe and fit a water filter to your supply. If you do, get one that filters out the undesirable elements but leaves in the calcium and magnesium. Jug filters aren't all that brilliant. All filters need regular cleaning or replacing to avoid bacteria build-up. Another way to avoid chemical pollutants in the water is to draw drinking water only from the cold tap and let it run for a couple of minutes before using. Hot water dissolves the undesirable elements, such as lead, much more easily than cold water does.

Which is best – hard water or soft water?

Hard water contains much more calcium and magnesium than soft water, and soft water contains more sodium than hard, so hard water is preferable. If you live in a soft water area be diligent about getting calcium and magnesium in your diet.

Which is best – tap water or bottled water?

The mineral content of bottled waters varies considerably. When choosing, look at the mineral content information and choose one that is, if possible, high in calcium and magnesium and low in sodium (less than 50mg per 100ml). Some mineral waters contain quite high levels of sodium.

There is no straightforward answer to the question which is best, as it depends upon the quality of the tap water and the variety of the mineral water or other bottled water that you choose.

The best answer is that whatever water you choose, it is going to do you much more good than being dehydrated!

Is it good to drink distilled water?

Whatever you may have heard to the contrary, I wouldn't drink distilled water. Certainly, the distillation process removes all the trace chemicals and pollutants from the water – but this includes calcium and magnesium and the other 'good for you' minerals. A filtering system that removes the nasties and leaves the goodies is better. Obviously, occasional distilled water won't do you any harm.

If I don't feel thirsty, surely I can't be dehydrated?

That isn't true. Usually, a conscious feeling of thirst is the body's last way of letting you know that it needs hydrating. It is its 'last resort' to nudge you to go and get a drink. Don't wait until you feel thirsty before drinking. Space water intake out regularly through the day, and take more water if you are exercising or are hot.

Omega Unit 12

Water Unit

One WATER UNIT consists of approximately SIX 8 to 10 fl oz (225ml to 300ml) glasses of water a day, spaced out evenly, as a minimum. (See chart on page 93 for your optimum amount.)

If slimming, drinking a glass before a meal is a simple way to dull the appetite. Sipping during a meal will also help.

Now I have introduced you to all twelve of the Omega Units. You will hear more about them in the next chapter, which pulls the complete Omega system together for you and presents the initial 14-day diet.

CHAPTER 6

The Omega Diet

Ω

Now it is time to put all the Omega Units together in the Omega system. This chapter will get you started with minimal fuss by providing a ready-designed 14-day diet for you to follow. This is followed by guidance on building your own diet by using the Omega Units as you wish.

The Omega Diet Q and A

How much will I be eating on my 12 units a day?

As already explained, you don't count calories as such under the Omega system, but if you are overweight and if you eat your 12 units a day, plus unlimited items as detailed below, you will lose weight because you will almost certainly be eating many fewer calories a day than you have been.

The 14-day diet that begins on page 108 divides the units up so that you have three meals and two small snacks a day, which is, I believe, the ideal way to eat. I strongly recommend that you do follow this set diet for at least two weeks so that you get into the Omega way of eating without having to think about your daily units. If you eat all you are allowed, you shouldn't feel hungry.

Once you are happy with the Omega way of eating you can go 'freeform' – choose your own menus from the foods you can eat within the 12 units – and continue to lose weight, as explained at the end of the chapter.

Once you are down to your ideal weight, you can go 'Omega Plus' – adding on extras to the basic units so that you are eating more, with more variety, all of which is explained in Chapter 8.

So if food isn't weighed or measured, how can I be sure I am reducing my calorie intake?

As I said at the outset, this is a diet for grown-ups and you need to exercise a modicum of commonsense when dishing up food for yourself. Portion control is up to you. Guidelines for the size of most of the units, should you want them, are given both at the end of Chapters 2 to 5 under the individual unit descriptions, and on page 102, under the heading 'Quick Guide to the Omega Units', but these will vary according to your sex, age, height, current weight, the amount of exercise you are doing and so on. The information and questionnaire below will help you to decide.

The main requisite is that you eat enough to satisfy your hunger, eat slowly, chew thoroughly, drink water – and stop eating when you feel full. If you have always been the kind of person who gets off on huge portions and a high-stacked plate, you are going to have to tame that urge and put a reasonable-sized portion on your plate.

If you finish your plateful and, having borne all the requisites above in mind, still feel genuinely hungry, then you should have a little more food, but preferably something different – add in an extra fruit unit, for instance, or some of your 'unlimited' yogurt.

If you find you are not losing weight on a reasonably regular basis while eating only your 12 units plus unlimiteds, then you are giving yourself overlarge portions and you should cut down. **It is always best to cut down portion sizes rather than cut down the number of times a day that you eat**.

If, however, you are losing weight too *quickly* while on the diet, you should increase your portion sizes, whether or not you feel hungry. For a discussion on how much weight you should expect to lose on this diet, see page 101.

Adjusting unit portion sizes to suit yourself

Ω *Your sex* Generally speaking, males have a higher percentage of body lean (muscle) than females, and because lean tissue is more metabolically active than fat, men can, as a rule, eat more than women even if all other factors (such as height and age) are the same. So if you are male, you may be able to increase portion sizes from the average guidelines given, which are based on the average female.

Ω *Your age* As a general rule, the younger you are, the more you need to eat to maintain your weight than an older person of the same sex, height, activity levels, etc. Therefore, even when slimming, you can eat more. So if you are under 30, you may be able to increase portion sizes from the averages given, which are based on people aged between 30 and 40.

  If you are over 40, you may need to cut down portion sizes slightly. The older you are over 40, the more likely it is that you may need to cut down in order to lose weight. If you aren't sure, go on the basic diet for two weeks – if you are losing weight well, you needn't cut down.

Ω *Your height* The taller you are, the more you can eat and still lose weight. Average heights are 5ft 10ins for males, and 5ft 5ins for females. If you are much under these heights you may need to cut down your portions; much taller, and you may need to eat more to satisfy your hunger.

Ω *Your current weight* The heavier you currently are, the more you can eat and still lose weight. The portion sizes given below are based on an average person wanting to lose a stone or so. If you have many stones to lose you will be able to increase your portion sizes. If you have only a few pounds to lose you may need to decrease portion sizes – or increase your activity levels (see next point).

Ω *Your activity levels* Highly active people need to eat more than sedentary people. The portion sizes are based on someone doing an average of four hours physical activity a week (say, a 20-minute walk, plus some stretching/toning exercises most days). When you're following the Omega Diet, I hope and suggest that you will exercise regularly and won't be sedentary; therefore, cutting back on portion sizes because you get no exercise won't be a necessity. For more on activity, see Chapter 8.

Portion Profile Questionnaire

To work out whether you are likely to need average, smaller or larger portions on the Omega Diet, go through the list of variables here, using the information on pages 98–9 to help you decide, and tick the appropriate box for each. Then add up your scores in each of the five ticked boxes to get your final result.

Sex	Male	+1				Female	−1
Age	Under 30	+1	30–40	0		Over 40	−1
Height *(males)*	6ft or over	+1	5ft 8 to 5ft 11	0		Under 5ft 8	−1
(females)	5ft 9 or over	+1	5ft 5 to 5ft 8	0		Under 5ft 5	−1
Weight to lose	Much over a stone	+1	About a stone	0		Half a stone or so	−1
Activity levels	Very active	+1	Moderately active	0		Sedentary	−1

What your score means

+5 to +3   You will almost definitely be able to increase your portion sizes.

+1 to +2   You may be able to have slightly larger portions than average.

0   You will probably do well on the average portion sizes listed with the units.

−1 to −2   You may have to decrease your portion sizes slightly in order to lose weight.

−3 to −5   You will almost definitely have to decrease your portions sizes in order to lose weight.

As an example, a male (+1) aged 45 (−1) of average height (0) with two stones to lose (+1), and with average activity levels (0), has a final score of +1, meaning that he may be able to have slightly larger portions than average.

As another example, a female (−1) aged 29 (+1) of lower than average height (−1) with three stones to lose (+1) and of average activity levels (0) has a final score of 0, meaning that she will do well on the average portion sizes listed with the units below.

HOWEVER, remember that it is best to be guided by your actual weight loss, rather than theory, throughout the 14-day diet and the freeform diet.

So how much weight am I likely to lose?

Losing weight is not an exact science, but I can certainly give you an estimate of what you can expect to lose.

If you scored a 'plus' result on the portion profile questionnaire on page 100, you can expect to lose up to 9lbs during the 14-day diet.

If you scored a neutral (average), you can expect to lose up to 7lbs during the 14-day diet.

If you scored a 'minus', you can expect to lose up to 5lbs during the 14-day diet.

HOWEVER, you must be aware that much of this initial weight loss will be fluid, not fat. This is because you are reducing calorie and carbohydrate intake, as well as salt. When you eat a high-calorie, high-carb diet, your body needs extra fluid to 'soak up' the food (think of blotting paper or a sponge). This is compounded by eating lots of salt, which many of you will have been doing – sodium (the major component of salt) also causes the body to retain more fluid, in order to dilute it to a safe level.

So changing over to the Omega Diet will cause a lot of body fluid to become 'surplus to requirements', and it will be excreted in the urine. You will find yourself going to the loo a lot more than you used to.

At least half of your initial weight loss during the two weeks will be fluid. Your body fluids will equalise again after this – that is, you won't lose any more, and then most of what weight you do lose will be fat, plus a little lean body tissue.

So after the 14 days are up, your weight loss will be less dramatic but more long-lasting, if you like. In the following weeks, you can expect a weight loss of between 1 and 3lbs a week, depending, again, upon your own body profile. If you are a 'minus' person, 1 to 1½lbs a week will be very good. If you are a 'plus' person, 2 to 3lbs a week will be very good.

In fact – if you are overweight, any regular weight loss is good, whether it is ½lb or 3lbs.

If, after the 14 days, you are losing more than 2lbs a week as a minus, or 3lbs a week as a plus, you should give yourself bigger portions. Do this gradually; you will soon find out how much is enough.

The Omega 14-day diet

You are almost ready now to get shopping for your first few days/week of the 14-day diet. But first do read the notes that follow – they are all very important to the success of your diet.

Understanding the units

Your Omega Diet consists of one of each of the 12 units a day (plus unlimiteds). You can start on the system almost straight away because the 14-day diet has done all the work for you in putting these units together into sensible, palatable menus.

You are already familiar with the units by reading about them in Chapters 2 to 5; however, you may want to consult the condensed guide that appears below from time to time.

For instance, if during the 14-day diet you come across a food item that you really can't eat (say, because of an allergy), use this potted guide to swap it for something you can eat WITHIN THE SAME UNIT GROUP.

Quick guide to the Omega Units

 PROTEIN UNIT Medium portion oily fish, large portion white fish, medium portion seafood, small portion organic lean meat, game, poultry, or Quorn.

NOTE: One to two 1,000mg omega-3 fish oil capsules are obligatory with each Protein Unit except oily fish.

 OIL UNIT Two tablespoons of oil a day. Either plain, good-quality *olive oil* (the preferred choice for high-temperature cooking), or the *oil blend* – olive oil blended with rapeseed oil (ratio of 100ml olive oil to 75ml rapeseed oil) for other cooking – or *salad oil blend* – a blend of one-third each rapeseed, walnut and groundnut oil for salads and cold use. The Oil Unit can be divided into two portions, used separately.

NUT UNIT Your unit is an average palmful. It will usually be a mix of fresh nuts in the ratio of 50% walnuts, 25% cashews and 25% hazelnuts. If nut mix is stated, use this. Occasionally within the 14-day diet other nuts are specified.

 SEED UNIT One heaped tablespoon seed mix, which is in the ratio of 50% pumpkin seeds, 25% linseeds and 25% sunflower seeds. If seed mix is stated, use this. Occasionally within the 14-day diet other seeds are specified.

C-FRUIT UNIT One medium to large portion (one large single fruit, two small fruits or one good bowlful of berry fruits) vitamin C-rich fruit – guava, blackcurrants, strawberries, papaya, kiwi fruit, oranges, clementines, nectarines, mango, grapefruit, raspberries, or a mixture of any of these. Eat raw.

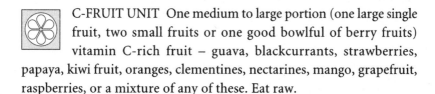 FRUIT-2 UNIT One medium to large portion of any other fresh fruit – apples, peaches, melon, cherries, red grapes, plums, pears (preferred choices). Mostly raw. Choose other fruits from time to time if you like (such as bananas).

OR one small to medium portion dried fruits – apricots, prunes, figs (preferred choices). Choose raisins and sultanas from time to time if you like. You can use them ready to eat or reconstituted without added sugar.

GREEN UNIT One large portion or two smaller portions (or more) of any fresh mid- to dark green vegetable or mixture of these – kale, spring greens, savoy or other dark cabbage, sprouts, spinach, green beans, broccoli (calabrese), purple sprouting broccoli, seaweed (preferred choices). Other choices are green beans, cos or other dark lettuce, broad beans, mangetout and peas.

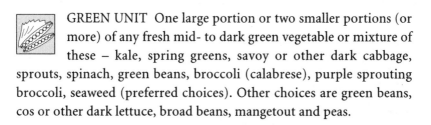 FLAME UNIT One medium to large portion of any fresh red, orange or yellow vegetable – red peppers, orange peppers, yellow peppers, tomatoes, carrots, orange-fleshed squash or pumpkin, swede, sweetcorn or a mixture of these.

PULSE UNIT One medium portion (about 150g cooked weight) pulses – dried beans, peas or lentils, such as Puy lentils, green lentils, kidney beans, cannellini beans, borlotti beans, butter beans, broad beans, baked beans, chickpeas, split peas, soya protein products such as tofu or TVP, lentil paté or hummus.

 QUALITY CARB UNIT This can be any one of the following.
Ω Up to 80g (about three slices) any wholegrain bread or one large wholewheat pitta or chapati.

Ω Up to four plain oatcakes or six dark rye crispbreads (such as Ryvita).

Ω One good portion (about 60g dry weight) wholegrain, such as brown basmati rice, wholewheat pasta, bulghar wheat, pot barley, oats, buckwheat, quinoa, millet or amaranth.

Ω One good portion (about 60g) wholegrain breakfast cereal, such as shredded wheat, old-fashioned porridge, All-Bran, muesli (the kind with no added sugar or salt), puffed wheat or Weetabix.

Ω One good portion (about 225g) new potatoes in their skins.

Ω One medium orange-fleshed sweet potato.

Ω OR 2 × half portions of any of these.

 CALCIUM UNIT At least 200g low-fat natural bio yogurt or calcium-enriched soya yogurt OR at least 300ml skimmed milk or calcium-enriched soya milk.

OR 2 × half portions of any of these.

Small tub of low-fat fromage frais, cottage cheese or half-fat Greek yogurt can be used occasionally.

 WATER UNIT Six to eight 8 to 10fl oz (225ml to 300ml) glasses of water a day, spaced out evenly. Before, with or just after meals or when exercising is ideal. See unlimiteds, below, for what you can add to this.

Unlimiteds

In addition to the Omega Units listed above, on the 14-day diet you can have a variety of items in unlimited quantities (use your common sense on the meaning of the word 'unlimited' – even healthy items such as water and carrots are toxic if you have too much of them). Here they are.

Ω *Salad items* All leafy green or red lettuces, cucumber, onions, celery, carrots, peppers, mushrooms, watercress, mustard and cress, rocket are included in this category.

Ω *Herbs and spices* This includes all fresh or dried herbs and spices, including garlic, chilli, ginger, parsley, basil, coriander and chives. Most herbs and spices (if fresh) have good health benefits, as you've seen in the preceding chapters, and you should try to incorporate them into your diet regularly.

Ω *Drinks* You can have herb and non-sweetened fruit teas, such as chamomile or rosehip; green tea; lemon juice (fresh), lime juice (fresh) and water.
NOTE: Keep ordinary tea and coffee for your first 14 days to a minimum and don't use your calcium allowance with either. Avoid all fizzy drinks and other sweet drinks even if they are low-calorie.

Ω *Condiments* These can be herbs and spices as above, including black pepper, tomato purée, passata, all vinegars and lemon and lime juice.

Ω *Miscellaneous* Low-fat natural bio yogurt is useful for a between-meal snack, especially if you add a few crudités from the unlimited salad list, a dash of lemon juice and some seasoning or herbs; or use it as a dressing ingredient.

Ω *Citrus fruit* You can have extra citrus fruit when you feel hungry or to add interest to a between-meal snack, over and above your ordinary C-Fruit Unit.

A NOTE ABOUT SALT: The Omega Diet is naturally quite low in salt as it avoids all the highly processed foods which are likely to contain most. Also the diet is high in potassium-rich fruits and vegetables, which balance out sodium, so you can use a little sea salt (which can be bought either in large flakes or ground more finely) in your cooking and in your dressings, and so on, but try to limit the amount you use. A diet high in salt is linked with high blood pressure and therefore with CHD and stroke. A diet low in sodium can reduce blood pressure considerably in people with high BP, and therefore reduce the risk of CHD and stroke.

Semi-limited condiments

During your 14 days you can use small amounts of a few other condiments to help add palatability and interest to your diet and your cooking. When I say 'small amounts', that is what I mean! Here they are.

- Ω *Soya sauce* Low in calories, soya sauce is also high in salt, so go fairly easily.
- Ω *Tahini* High in calories but healthy, this sesame seed paste adds flavour to oil dressings, hummus, casseroles and so on.
- Ω *Worcestershire sauce* This is low-calorie, and high on flavour, but also quite salty.
- Ω *Honey* A little runny honey won't do you any harm, especially if it is organic. But limit yourself to the odd small drizzle.
- Ω *Dark brown sugar* A pinch of this added to dressings or stir fries is good. Sugar used for any other purpose isn't allowed!
- Ω *Sundried tomato paste* Full of beta-carotene and rich flavour, this makes a good addition to soups, casseroles and so on, but it can be oily and therefore high in calories.

The importance of organic

Whenever possible, please buy all your food and drink organic. Why choose a healthy, natural diet for yourself like the Omega Diet, and then spoil it by buying less than natural food which has been treated with pesticides, or preservatives, may contain GM ingredients, and so on? For more on organic eating and buying, see Chapter 8.

The importance of eating regularly

The Omega Diet allows you three meals and two small snacks a day and you should space these out as evenly as you can. (If you want to refresh your memory about why, read about blood sugar levels on pages 24 and 76–7.) If you want to, you can move the evening meal to lunchtime, and vice versa.

The importance of variety

By following the 14-day diet as it is laid out, you will be getting all your units and you will be getting a wide variety of different items within those units. This is an important lesson to learn. Healthy eating isn't just about the right major nutrients but about getting all the vitamins and minerals and phytochemicals which only a varied diet can provide.

Don't be afraid to add any of the unlimited items to your diet. These add colour, texture and flavour and help to fill your plate up, especially if the portion questionnaire revealed that you should pay extra attention to portion control. Many of the items, especially the salads, herbs, spices and yogurt, provide valuable additional nutrition, too.

Shopping for your diet

It is a good idea to go through your larder and fridge before you do anything else, and chuck out any items which may tempt you off your Omega Diet. You also need to make some space for all the great foods that you *will* be eating.

Then make a list and shop for your diet. Try to do all your shopping for non-perishables for the whole two weeks, then shop for fresh fruit and vegetables every three days or so. Store as much as you can in the fridge. Stale produce quickly loses its vitamin C, texture and flavour.

Fish and meat should be bought and used the same day, or bought really fresh and frozen – or you could buy top-quality already frozen.

Don't forget that if food isn't stuffed full of preservatives, it won't keep as long. This is particularly true of organic bread (slice and freeze it if necessary) and organic yogurt.

Water

Don't forget to drink water with every meal and in between so that you get your total daily unit.

Now it is time to start . . . (The recipes referred to begin on page 131.)

Day One

BREAKFAST

Medium portion low-fat bio yogurt with 1 satsuma
and 1 kiwi fruit chopped and stirred in

MIDMORNING SNACK

Nut mix

LUNCH

1 portion Hummus (see recipe, page 136) and
sliced red and yellow peppers and red onion,
stir-fried in a little olive oil until soft, all served on
top of one slice of dark rye bread or with one
mini wholewheat pitta
1 apple

AFTERNOON SNACK

Medium portion low-fat bio yogurt
1 satsuma

EVENING MEAL

1 portion Rainbow Trout Fillets with Tapenade
(see recipe, page 145)
Green beans and broccoli
½ portion brown rice

Day Two

BREAKFAST

1 Weetabix
1 large dessert pear or peach, chopped
Skimmed milk or soya milk to cover

MIDMORNING SNACK

1 orange
Nut mix

LUNCH

1 portion Rice and Beans Salad
(see recipe, page 139)
Salad leaves to garnish

AFTERNOON SNACK

Low-fat natural fromage frais
Teaspoon runny honey

EVENING MEAL

1 small portion roast, baked or grilled organic
chicken (skin removed)
Lightly cooked spring greens, peas
Carrots
1 to 2 omega-3 fish oil capsules

Day Three

BREAKFAST

Small portion porridge made with traditional
porridge oats, and half skimmed milk
(or soya milk) and half water sprinkled with
1 portion seed mix
1 orange

MIDMORNING SNACK

Medium portion low-fat natural bio yogurt
Teaspoon runny honey

LUNCH

1 portion Puy Lentil and Squash Soup
(see recipe, page 131)

AFTERNOON SNACK

1 apple
Nut mix

EVENING MEAL

Large portion white fish of choice, baked, steamed
or grilled
Broccoli
Salad of sliced tomatoes, spring onions and rocket
leaves all tossed in 2 tablespoons French
Dressing (see recipe, page 156)
½ portion brown rice
1 to 2 omega-3 fish oil capsules

Day Four

BREAKFAST

Medium portion low-fat natural fromage frais
Kiwi fruit and raspberries

MIDMORNING SNACK

Nut mix

LUNCH

1 portion Salade Nicoise (see recipe, page 140)
1 slice organic wholemeal or rye bread

AFTERNOON SNACK

Seed mix
Medium portion low-fat natural bio yogurt
Teaspoon runny honey

EVENING MEAL

1 portion Spicy Stuffed Peppers
   (see recipe, page 146)
Side salad of cos lettuce, watercress and rocket
½ portion bulghar wheat
1 slice melon or 1 apple

Day Five

BREAKFAST

1 shredded wheat with plenty of skimmed milk or
soya milk to cover
Sliced strawberries or kiwi fruit

MIDMORNING SNACK

Handful shelled almonds (skins on)

LUNCH

1 portion Orange and Rice Salad
(see recipe, page 140)
Watercress garnish

AFTERNOON SNACK

Medium portion low-fat natural bio yogurt
2 plums or handful red grapes

EVENING MEAL

1 portion salmon, plainly cooked
(such as grilled or baked)
Broccoli, green beans
1 portion Black Bean Salsa (see recipe, page 141)

Day Six

BREAKFAST

Medium portion low-fat natural bio yogurt with
1 portion orange-fleshed melon OR 1 peach
chopped in and topped with seed mix

MIDMORNING SNACK

Nut mix

LUNCH

1 portion Spinach, Watercress and Pea Soup
(see recipe, page 132)
½ portion Spicy Tofu Dip (see recipe, page 136)
and ¼ portion Hummus (see recipe, page 136)
Carrot and celery crudites

AFTERNOON SNACK

1 orange

EVENING MEAL

1 portion Lemon Lamb Kebabs with Tzatziki
(see recipe, page 151)
Pitta
Mixed green salad
1 to 2 omega-3 fish oil capsules

Day Seven

BREAKFAST

1 portion Apricot and Apple Milkshake
(see recipe, page 156)

MIDMORNING SNACK

Handful walnuts

LUNCH

1 portion Panzanella (see recipe, page 142)
1 portion grilled fresh sardines

AFTERNOON SNACK

1 kiwi fruit, 1 clementine

EVENING MEAL

1 portion Chickpea, Spinach and Aubergine Harissa
(see recipe, page 147)
½ portion brown rice

Day Eight

BREAKFAST

Medium portion low-fat natural fromage frais
Dried Fruit Breakfast Compote
    (see recipe, page 155)
Seed mix

MIDMORNING SNACK

1 orange
Medium portion low-fat natural bio yogurt

LUNCH

1 portion Lentil Paté (see recipe, page 137)
Large mixed salad tossed in 1 portion French
    Dressing (see recipe, page 156)
1 slice rye bread

AFTERNOON SNACK

Celery crudités with ½ portion Spicy Tofu Dip
    (see recipe, page 136)
Nut mix

EVENING MEAL

1 portion Chicken and Pasta Casserole
    (see recipe, page 152)
Brussels sprouts, kale
1 to 2 omega-3 fish oil capsules

Day Nine

BREAKFAST

Medium portion low-fat natural bio yogurt
1 orange
Seed mix

MIDMORNING SNACK

Handful Brazil nuts

LUNCH

1 portion Split Pea, Mint and Vegetable Soup
(see recipe, page 132)
1 slice wholewheat or rye bread

AFTERNOON SNACK

Handful red grapes
Spoonful low-fat natural bio yogurt

EVENING MEAL

1 portion Catalan Tuna with Tomato Sauce
(see recipe, page 145)
Green beans and broccoli with a little oil blend
drizzled over

Day Ten

BREAKFAST

1 shredded wheat with skimmed milk or soya milk
to cover
Mixed red berry fruits
Seed mix

MIDMORNING SNACK

Nut mix

LUNCH

Medium portion smoked peppered trout with
lemon juice
Large mixed salad including some dark green
leaves, such as baby spinach, watercress,
and rocket, with 1 to 2 tablespoons French
Dressing (see recipe, page 156)

AFTERNOON SNACK

1 mango, papaya or nectarine

EVENING MEAL

1 portion Mexican Chilli (see recipe, page 148)
$\frac{1}{2}$ portion brown rice

Day Eleven

BREAKFAST

1 small bowl porridge made with traditional oats,
  half skimmed milk or soya milk and half water
1 apple

MIDMORNING SNACK

Medium portion low-fat natural bio yogurt
Teaspoon runny honey

LUNCH

1 portion Fruit, Nut and Pasta Salad
  (see recipe, page 142)
Salad leaves

AFTERNOON SNACK

Celery crudités with Spicy Tofu Dip
  (see recipe, page 136)

EVENING MEAL

1 medium portion salmon, plainly cooked and
  served on a bed of cooked brown or Puy lentils,
  drizzled with 1 to 2 tablespoons oil blend
Green beans
Chargrilled red peppers

Day Twelve

BREAKFAST

Medium portion low-fat natural bio yogurt
Sliced strawberries and kiwi fruit
Seed mix

MIDMORNING SNACK

Nut mix

LUNCH

1 portion Carrot and Tomato Soup
  (see recipe, page 133)
1 portion Smoked Mackerel Paté
  (see recipe, page 138),
Salad leaves
1 slice rye bread

AFTERNOON SNACK

1 small banana
Glass of skimmed or soya milk

EVENING MEAL

1 portion Falafel Patties (see recipe, page 149)
New potatoes, scrubbed and tossed with
  1 tablespoon olive oil and seasoning and baked
  until tender at 200°C
Large mixed salad with 1 tablespoon French
  Dressing (see recipe, page 156)
Peas

Day Thirteen

BREAKFAST
1 portion Apricot and Apple Milkshake
(see recipe, page 156)

MIDMORNING SNACK
Medium portion low-fat natural bio yogurt
Seed mix

LUNCH
1 portion Tabbouleh (see recipe, page 143)
1 portion Hummus (see recipe, page 136)
Red pepper and carrot crudités

AFTERNOON SNACK
1 orange

EVENING MEAL
1 portion herring or trout fillets, baked or grilled
1 portion Classic Waldorf Salad
(see recipe, page 144)
Broccoli

Day Fourteen

BREAKFAST

Medium portion low-fat natural bio yogurt
Small portion no added sugar or salt muesli
Chopped apple

MIDMORNING SNACK

Handful red grapes

LUNCH

1 portion Italian Three Bean Salad
   (see recipe, page 144)
Salad leaves

AFTERNOON SNACK

Carrot and celery crudités with Spicy Tofu Dip
   (see recipe, page 136)

EVENING MEAL

1 portion Pork and Cashews with Noodles
   (see recipe, page 153)

NEXT

Either repeat the diet if you like, or move on to the Omega Freeform
Diet as explained next (which is still for weight loss but allows you to
devise your own diet), or, if you simply want to maintain your weight
now, move on to Chapter 8.

The Omega Freeform Diet

To lose weight on foods that you enjoy in combinations that you want, all you need to do is remember the 12 units, get one of each daily, plus unlimiteds items – and you can carry on dieting as long as you like, down to your ideal weight.

Here are some guidelines to help you plan your diet successfully.

Just count to 12!

To help you keep track of your daily units, use the blank charts at the back of the book on pages 176 to 180 (cut them out if you want to). When all the spaces are filled up each day, you've used all your units.

To remind you again, your units are:

Protein	Green
Oil	Flame
Nut	Pulse
Seed	Quality Carb
C-Fruit	Calcium
Fruit-2	Water

Don't miss out any of the units on any day of your diet.

You can split your Oil, Quality Carb and Calcium Units up into halves if you like, but don't tick the space until you have eaten both halves.

Space it out!

Don't forget to space your units out throughout the day so that you eat regularly. It doesn't matter which units you get at which meal or snack, but you will find out, as the days progress, which combinations please you most.

The only exception to this is that you should aim to have a calcium or a protein or a pulse at the three main meals of the day – breakfast, lunch and your evening meal. By following this rule you won't be tempted to eat nothing but, say, a piece of fruit at lunchtime – and then wonder why you don't feel full enough.

Here is a good breakdown of how you might use your units most days:

Breakfast: 2 to 3 units, including calcium and a fruit.
Lunch: 2 to 4 units, using a protein or pulse and at least one veg.
Evening meal: 3 to 4 units, using a protein or pulse and at least ½ Quality Carb Unit.
Two between-meal snacks a day of 1 to 2 units each.
PLUS plenty of *unlimiteds*, and water with each meal or snack and in between meals.

Keep it varied!

Just as with the 14-day diet, it is important that you have a wide variety of items in your diet – both to ensure you get the complete range of nutrients that each unit encompasses, and so that you don't get bored. Make a note of meals that you particularly enjoy. Look out for recipes and meal ideas in magazines and books that will fit in with the Omega way of eating. And don't be frightened to cook – all the recipes in this book are simple.

Of course, you can take any meals and snacks from the 14-day set diet and use them in your freeform diet. The list of meal ideas that follows will help you to broaden your diet, too.

However, don't forget that if you are rushed or don't like cooking, there is no harm in keeping your diet simple sometimes. A very fresh fillet of fish, plainly cooked with nothing more than a dressed mixed salad, makes a delicious meal – and is ideal if you've already used up your Quality Carb Unit.

Or pasta dressed in nothing more than olive oil and tapenade and served with a tomato and basil salad makes a great meal, especially if you've used up your Protein and Pulse Units.

If you are cutting the junk foods out of your diet – simple things will taste all the better.

How are you doing?

You will know if you are doing well on the freeform diet if you are losing weight steadily. Remember, if you are losing weight too FAST, increase portion sizes and/or increase the size of your Quality Carb Unit. If you are losing weight too SLOWLY, reduce portion sizes of all the units (except water) by a very small amount and try to take more exercise.

Once you no longer want to lose weight, turn to Chapter 8.

A word about packed lunches

Some of you may find that you have problems at lunchtime if you are used to eating in cafeterias or usually purchase a takeaway. Many of the lunches in the list below are suitable for packing and taking to work. All you may need is a wide-necked vacuum flask (for soups) or a secure insulated plastic box (for salads and sandwiches), plus a good-quality set of disposable utensils.

Within the list are some ready-to-eat items that you can buy in the shops. We all need a quick takeaway now and then.

You will find more information about eating the Omega way during the normal course of your life in Chapter 8.

Meal ideas for the Freeform Diet

NOTE: Within some of the meal suggestions, whether you choose a whole or a half Quality Carb Unit will depend upon whether you want to save any carb for the rest of the day. You could even omit the Quality Carb altogether (say, because you want it at a different meal in the day).

NOTE: Green salad only makes a Green Unit if it is very large and contains lots of dark green leaves and/or other green veg such as green peppers or green beans. Other salad only makes a Flame Unit if it contains the equivalent of at least one large tomato or one medium red or orange pepper.

Lunches

Ω *Salad:* cooked green lentils mixed with chopped spring onions, tomato, crisp lettuce, cucumber and artichoke hearts (optional) tossed with 1 portion French Dressing (see page 156). (1 Pulse Unit, ½ Oil Unit) Serve with optional rye bread. (½ or 1 Quality Carb Unit)

Ω *Salad:* Tuna, fresh or canned in olive oil, drained, flaked and served with canned, drained butterbeans or cannellini beans, sliced tomato, sliced yellow peppers, sliced red onion and parsley, tossed with 1 portion French Dressing. (1 Protein Unit, ½ Pulse Unit, 1 Flame Unit, ½ Oil Unit)

Ω *Salad:* 1 chicken breast, grilled, cooled and sliced with segmented orange; 1 Little Gem lettuce, sliced into wedges; sliced red onion and plenty of walnuts, all tossed in 1 portion French Dressing. (1 Protein Unit, 1 C-Fruit Unit, 1 Nut Unit, ½ Oil Unit)

Ω *Salad:* Peeled prawns surrounded by slices of ripe canteloupe melon and pineapple; served with a slice of wholewheat bread. (1 protein unit, 1 Fruit-2 Unit, ½ Quality Carb Unit)

Ω *Salad:* Dressed crab combined with light soya sauce, crushed garlic, lime juice, coriander leaves, half a fresh red chilli, de-seeded and chopped, plus a little salad oil blend, served on crisp mixed salad leaves, 1 omega-3 fish oil capsule. (1 Protein Unit, ½ Oil Unit)

Ω *Salad:* 1 rollmop herring, cut into chunks and mixed with some grated beetroot, some ruby chard, a small red eating apple, diced, and some well-seasoned low-fat bio yogurt mixed with a little lemon juice, a pinch of caster sugar and a pinch of creamed horseradish. (1 Protein Unit)

Ω *Soup:* Ready-to-eat fresh soup from supermarket – lentil and vegetable – and 1 slice rye bread. (1 Pulse Unit, ½ Quality Carb Unit)

Ω *Soup:* 1 portion fresh chilled watercress soup; 1 portion Lentil Paté (see recipe, page 137) with 1 wholemeal roll or 3 rye crispbreads. (1 Green Unit, 1 Pulse Unit, ½ Quality Carb Unit)

Ω *Soup:* 1 portion fresh chilled carrot and coriander soup; 1 wholemeal roll. (1 Flame Unit, ½ Quality Carb Unit, ½ Calcium Unit) Avoid soups containing cream. Skimmed milk is okay – check ingredients.

Ω *Soup:* 1 small can butterbeans in water, well drained and rinsed, and pureéd with chopped softened onion, 2 to 3 cooked new potatoes and 200ml skimmed milk or calcium-enriched soya milk, seasoned and heated. (1 Pulse Unit, ½ Quality Carb Unit, 1 Calcium Unit)

Ω *Toast:* Large slice wholemeal toast drizzled with a little oil blend and topped with a portion of low-salt baked beans in tomato sauce OR 1 portion Boston Baked Beans (see recipe, page 135). (1 Quality Carb Unit, 1 Pulse Unit, ½ Oil Unit)

Ω *Toast:* Large slice wholemeal toast drizzled with a little oil blend and topped with several fresh grilled sardines, well seasoned, plus lemon wedges. (1 Quality Carb Unit, ½ Oil Unit, 1 Protein Unit)

Ω *Paté:* Portion Smoked Mackerel Paté (see recipe, page 138) with mixed salad, balsamic vinegar dressing, 3 rye crispbreads. (1 Protein Unit, ½ Quality Carb Unit)

Ω *Hummus:* Portion Hummus (see recipe, page 136), 1 wholewheat pitta or 3 rye crispbreads, large dark green mixed leaf salad. (1 Pulse Unit, ½ Quality Carb Unit, 1 Green Unit, 1 Oil Unit)

Ω *Tofu:* 1 portion Marinated Tofu (see recipe, page 157), fried in a little olive oil or oil blend until golden and served on 1 slice rye bread with 1 large field mushroom, brushed with olive oil and baked, seasoned well, and a side salad. (1 Pulse Unit, ½ Oil Unit, ½ Quality Carb Unit)

Ω *Burger:* 1 TVP (soya mince) vegetarian burger, lightly fried in olive oil or oil blend and served with a large mixed salad, including watercress and baby spinach, and a little French Dressing. (1 Pulse Unit, 1 Oil Unit, 1 Green Unit)

Ω *Sausages:* 2 TVP (soya mince) sausages, dry-fried in a non-stick pan and served with a large tomato and onion salad with 1 portion French Dressing. (1 Pulse Unit, 1 Flame Unit, ½ Oil Unit)

Ω *Pitta:* 1 portion lentil dhal (from deli or out of can from health food shop) served with 1 wholewheat pitta or chapati and a mixed salad. (1 Pulse Unit, 1 Quality Carb Unit)

Ω *Ready meal:* 1 ready made salad: St Michael New York Deli Pasta Salad (205g) (1 Quality Carb Unit, ½ Oil Unit, 1 Nut Unit)

Ω *Ready meal:* 1 ready made filled flatbread, chicken and pesto variety. (1 Quality Carb Unit, 1 Protein Unit, ½ Oil Unit)

Main Meals

Ω *Fish:* 1 medium trout, baked and served with a handful of lightly toasted almonds, lemon wedges, broccoli and baked tomatoes. (1 Protein Unit, 1 Nut Unit, 1 Green Unit, 1 Flame Unit)

Ω *Fish:* 1 medium herring, baked or grilled and served with a sauce made from 2 tablespoons half-fat Greek yogurt mixed with a little wholegrain French mustard and seasoning; green beans. (1 Protein Unit, 1 Green Unit)

Ω *Fish:* 5 or 6 medium fresh sardines, grilled and served with 1 tablespoon toasted pine nuts, 1 dessertspoon warmed redcurrant jelly; large dark green leafy salad. (1 Protein Unit, 1 Seed Unit, 1 Green Unit)

Ω *Fish:* 1 portion white fish fillet of choice, marinated for an hour in lemon juice, oil blend, crushed garlic, finely chopped onion and a dash of white wine and seasoning, then fried in the marinade in a non-stick pan; brown rice, peas; omega-3 fish oil capsule. (1 Protein Unit, 1 Quality Carb Unit, 1 Green Unit, ½ Oil Unit)

Ω *Fish:* 1 whole bass or tilapia or salmon fillet, topped with finely shredded fresh chilli, ginger and spring onions, well seasoned and steamed; brown rice, mangetout. (1 Protein Unit, 1 Quality Carb Unit, 1 Green Unit)

Ω *Fish:* Monkfish fillet, cubed, and peeled prawns stir-fried with chopped ginger, garlic and chilli and a selection of green and flame vegetables in a little olive oil, with soya sauce added to taste; wholewheat noodles; omega-3 fish oil capsule. (1 Protein Unit, 1 Green Unit, 1 Flame Unit, 1 Quality Carb Unit)

Ω *Fish:* 1 swordfish or tuna steak, grilled, large dark green salad; grilled tomatoes. (1 Protein Unit, 1 Green Unit, 1 Flame Unit)

Ω *Lentils:* 1 portion Mushroom and Lentil Hotpot (see recipe, page 150); savoy cabbage. (1 Pulse Unit, ¼ Oil Unit, 1 Green Unit)

Ω *Tofu:* Portion Marinated Tofu (see recipe, page 157) cubed and threaded on to kebab stick with cubed red peppers and red onion, brushed with some marinade and grilled until golden; bulghar wheat; broccoli. (1 Pulse Unit, 1 Flame Unit, 1 Quality Carb Unit, 1 Green Unit)

Ω *Tofu and pasta:* Mix cooked wholewheat pasta shapes with cooked chopped green beans and mangetout and toss with a portion of cubed and grilled Marinated Tofu (see recipe, page 157), salad oil blend, seasoning and some crushed cumin and coriander seeds. (1 Quality Carb Unit, 1 Pulse Unit, 1 Green Unit, ½ Oil Unit)

Ω *Meat:* 1 portion Mediterranean Meatballs in a Rich Red Sauce (see recipe, page 154); wholewheat spaghetti; large dark green side salad with 1 portion French Dressing (see recipe, page 156); omega-3 fish oil capsule. (1 Oil Unit, 1 Protein Unit, 1 Flame Unit, 1 Quality Carb Unit, 1 Green Unit)

Ω *Meat:* 1 small to medium fillet steak or venison steak, grilled, with a large tomato and rocket salad dressed in 1 portion French Dressing. (1 Protein Unit, 1 Flame Unit, ½ Oil Unit)

Ω *Chicken:* 1 chicken breast, cut into four and arranged on a baking dish with quartered tomato, red onion chunks and courgette slices, all brushed with olive oil, seasoned and baked for 40 minutes or until cooked through. (1 Protein Unit, 1 Flame Unit)

Ω *Chicken:* 1 chicken breast, skinned, cut into four and marinated in lemon juice, 1 tablespoon olive oil, chopped parsley and crushed garlic, baked or grilled until cooked and served with green beans and spinach. (1 Protein Unit, 1 Green Unit, ½ Oil Unit)

Ω *Pasta:* 1 portion wholewheat pasta, cooked and tossed in 2 tablespoons salad oil blend into which you have pounded 1 portion nut mix, seasoning, crushed garlic and parsley; large mixed salad. (1 Quality Carb Unit, 1 Oil Unit, 1 Nut Unit, 1 Green Unit)

Ω *Pasta:* 1 portion wholewheat pasta, cooked and tossed with 1 portion mixed seafood (available ready prepared, frozen or chilled), and 1 portion tomato sauce (good quality ready made, or home-made using the recipe on page 145 but omitting the tuna) ; large mixed dark leaf green salad. (1 Quality Carb Unit, 1 Protein Unit, 1 Flame Unit, 1 Green Unit, ½ Oil Unit)

Ω *Pasta:* 1 portion wholewheat pasta, cooked and tossed with 1 portion of Bolognese sauce made from TVP (soya) mince simmered with tomato sauce; large dark green salad. (1Quality Carb Unit, 1 Pulse Unit, 1 Flame Unit, 1 Green Unit, ½ Oil Unit)

Ω *Ready Meal:* 1 Weight Watchers' Vegetable Ravioli in Tomato Sauce (1 Quality Carb Unit, I Flame Unit)

Ω *Ready Meal:* 1 Marks and Spencer's Salmon in Soy and Ginger Sauce (1 Protein Unit, ½ Oil Unit)

Ω *Ready Meal:* 1 Birds Eye Healthy Options Glazed Chicken (1 Protein Unit, ½ Quality Carb Unit)

Ω *Ready Meal:* 1 Tesco Vegetable Masala Rice Bowl (1 Quality Carb Unit)

CHAPTER 7

The Omega Recipes

All recipes serve 2 unless otherwise stated.
The Omega Units each recipe contains PER
PORTION is stated above each ingredients list.

Soups and hot snacks

Puy Lentil and Squash Soup

Providing: *1 Pulse Unit,*
1 Flame Unit, ¼ Oil Unit

150g (dry weight) Puy lentils
1 tablespoon olive oil
1 medium onion, finely chopped
1 stick celery, chopped
1 clove garlic, chopped
500ml vegetable stock
2 medium carrots, chopped
250g butternut squash, peeled, de-seeded and cut into chunks
2 tablespoons fresh chopped parsley
Little sea salt
Black pepper

Wash the lentils in a colander. Heat the oil in a saucepan and add the onion, celery and garlic and cook, stirring, for 2 to 3 minutes. Add the lentils, stock, carrot and squash and simmer for up to an hour until all the vegetables and the lentils are tender, adding half the parsley in the last few minutes of cooking. Remove from heat and when it has cooled slightly, pour half the soup into an electric blender if you have one and pureé, then return to the pan and stir in well. Add salt to taste and the pepper, and serve reheated with the remaining parsley sprinkled over.

○ If you don't have a blender you can serve the soup as is.
○ Add a level teaspoon of ground cumin with the garlic for a warmer soup.

131

Spinach, Watercress and Pea Soup

Providing: *¼ Oil Unit, 1 Green Unit,*
½ Quality Carb Unit

 200g new potatoes
 400ml vegetable stock
 1 tablespoon olive oil
 1 small to medium onion, chopped
 1 clove garlic, chopped
 200g fresh spinach, washed and any large stalks removed
 75g frozen or fresh, tender small peas
 1 bunch watercress, washed and most of stalks removed
 Sea salt
 Black pepper

Peel the potatoes and cut into small chunks. Bring the stock to the boil in a saucepan, add the potatoes and simmer. Meanwhile, heat the oil in a non-stick frying pan and gently sauté the onion until soft and transparent, adding the garlic towards the end of the frying time and making sure it doesn't brown. Stir the spinach into the frying pan to wilt slightly, then tip the whole lot into the saucepan with the potatoes, the peas and the watercress. Simmer, covered, for 20 more minutes or until the potatoes are tender, and then allow to cool for a few minutes before puréeing for no more than a few seconds in an electric blender so you have a nicely amalgamated but still very textured soup.

Return to the pan, taste and add a little sea salt and some black pepper. Reheat and serve garnished with extra watercress if liked.

Split Pea, Mint and Vegetable Soup

Provides: *¼ Oil Unit, 1 Pulse Unit,*
½ Quality Carb Unit

 75g dried split green peas
 1 medium potato (about 200g)

400ml vegetable stock
1 tablespoon olive oil
1 clove garlic, chopped
1 large leek, washed and chopped
1 large stick celery, chopped
75g broccoli, cut into florets
Handful chopped fresh mint
Sea salt
Black pepper
Whole mint leaves

Wash the split peas. Peel the potato and cut it into chunks. Put the stock in a saucepan, and add the peas and potatoes. Bring to a simmer and cover. Meanwhile, heat the oil in a non-stick saucepan and sauté the garlic, leek and celery for a few minutes until slightly softened, then add everything to the saucepan along with the broccoli. Simmer for 30 minutes or until the split peas are tender, then allow to cool for a few minutes and pureé half of the soup in an electric blender along with the chopped mint. Return the pureé to the saucepan, stir in well and add a little more stock if the soup seems too thick. Taste for seasoning, adding sea salt and pepper. Reheat and serve garnished with fresh mint leaves.

Carrot and Tomato Soup

Provides: ¼ *Oil Unit, 1 Flame Unit*, ½ *Quality Carb Unit*

1 tablespoon olive oil
1 clove garlic, chopped
1 medium onion, chopped
1 teaspoon ground cumin
1 teaspoon ground coriander seed
2 medium to large carrots, peeled and chopped
2 large tasty fresh tomatoes, skinned and chopped
350ml vegetable stock

1 bay leaf
Sea salt
Black pepper
Fresh coriander leaves (optional)
2 dessertspoons Spicy Tofu Dip (see recipe, page 136)

Heat the olive oil gently in a saucepan and sauté the onion and garlic until they are becoming soft. Add the cumin, coriander and carrots and stir for a minute until you can smell the spices. Add the tomatoes, stock and bay leaf, bring to a simmer and cover. Simmer for 20 minutes or until the carrots are soft, then cool for a few minutes and pureé in a blender, adding salt and pepper to taste. Reheat and serve garnished with coriander leaves and Spicy Tofu Dip.

Red Pepper and Basil Soup

Provides: ½ *Oil Unit, 1 Flame Unit*

2 red peppers, de-seeded and sliced
1 tablespoon cooking oil blend (see page 34)
300ml passata (sieved tomatoes)
Standard supermarket pot fresh basil
2 cloves garlic
Sea salt
Black pepper
1 tablespoon olive oil

Brush the peppers with some of the oil blend and grill or bake them until small areas of the pepper skin are becoming charred, then pop into an electric blender with the rest of the oil blend and the passata. Blend until smooth. Meanwhile, take most of the fresh basil, destalk and pound in a pestle and mortar with the garlic, salt, pepper and olive oil until you have a thick sauce. Stir this into the soup, heat gently in a saucepan, check for seasoning and then serve garnished with the remaining basil leaves.

Boston Baked Beans

Provides: *½ Oil Unit, 1 Pulse Unit,*
1 Flame Unit

125g dried haricot beans
2 tablespoons cooking oil blend (see page 34)
1 medium onion, finely chopped
1 good stick celery, chopped
2 medium carrots, chopped small
1 tablespoon dark treacle
1 dessertspoon brown sugar
200ml passata
1 tablespoon sundried tomato paste
1 teaspoon wholegrain French mustard
1 dessertspoon soya sauce
50ml stout
Sea salt
Black pepper

Soak the beans overnight, drain, cover with cold water in a saucepan, bring to a boil for 10 minutes, then turn heat down and simmer for 1 hour or until tender. Drain. Put the beans in a casserole dish with the rest of the ingredients, stirring well. Cover with a tight-fitting lid and cook in the oven for 2 hours at 150°C or until everything is tender and you have a rich sauce. (It is a good idea to check halfway through cooking – if the beans look too dry, add a little boiling water and stir.) Before serving, check for seasoning and adjust as necessary.

○ You can use pre-cooked haricot beans if you like, in which case you will need 400g ready cooked beans.
○ If you don't want to use stout, add some vegetable stock, red wine or tomato juice.
○ These beans are an excellent change from canned baked beans, served on wholemeal or rye toast, or they can be served as a main meal with brown rice or with baked sweet potatoes.

Dips, pureés, patés

Hummus

Provides: *1 Oil Unit, 1 Pulse Unit, 1 Seed Unit*

1 can ready cooked chickpeas in water, drained, water reserved
2 tablespoons tahini paste
2 good garlic cloves, crushed
4 tablespoons olive oil
Juice of 1 lemon
Sea salt
Black pepper

Put all the ingredients in an electric blender and blend until you have a thick pureé. Check seasoning, adding extra salt, pepper and lemon juice as necessary. If the hummus is too thick or you have trouble blending it, add some of the chickpea water until you have the right consistency. Put in an airtight container in the fridge until needed (it will keep for a few days) or serve immediately.

Spicy Tofu Dip

Provides: *½ Pulse Unit, ½ Oil Unit*

100g silken tofu
2 tablespoons salad oil blend (see page 34)
1 teaspoon French mustard
1 dessertspoon lemon juice
1 jalapeño chilli, de-seeded and finely chopped
Sea salt
Black pepper

Blend all the ingredients in a blender or with a fork in a bowl. Taste for seasoning, spoon into an airtight container and refrigerate until needed. This will keep for a few days.

o Omit the chilli if you prefer. Try other flavourings, such as chopped dill or spring onions, a little curry paste or crushed garlic. For the maintenance diet, some feta cheese can be crumbled into it.

o For a non-dairy mayonnaise, the dip can be thinned down as required with extra oil/lemon juice.

Lentil Paté

Provides: ½ *Pulse Unit*

50g Puy lentils (dry weight)
250ml vegetable stock
1 shallot, finely chopped
2 sage leaves, finely chopped
1 tablespoon tomato pureé
Sea salt
Black pepper

Simmer the lentils and onion in the stock on a very low heat, uncovered, until they are tender – about 30 to 40 minutes. Then add the rest of the ingredients, mix well and blend in an electric blender until you have a smooth paté. Check seasoning and serve.

o This paté is good served with toast or rye crispbreads. You can also thin it down by using extra stock, to make a spread for sandwiches on your maintenance diet or for a dip which you can serve with crudités.

Smoked Mackerel Paté

Provides: *1 Protein Unit*

2 smoked mackerel fillets (about 225g in all)
1 small pot natural low-fat bio yogurt (150ml)
2 tablespoons tomato pureé
Dash of soya sauce
1 tablespoon chopped fresh parsley
Sea salt
Black pepper

Flake the mackerel in a bowl using a fork. Add the yogurt, tomato pureé, soya sauce, parsley and seasoning. Combine until the mixture looks properly amalgamated. Cover and chill, serve. Use within 36 hours.

○ An electric blender doesn't tend to work well with this recipe.

Broad Bean Dip

Provides: *½ Green Unit, ½ Oil Unit*

175g shelled tender young broad beans
1 large garlic clove, crushed
1 level tablespoon freshly grated Parmesan cheese
2 tablespoons salad oil blend (see page 34)
Juice of ¼ lemon
Black pepper
Sea salt, if necessary

Cook the beans lightly in boiling salted water for 3 minutes or until just tender. Drain well. Put all ingredients in a blender and blend until smooth.

Salads

Rice and Beans Salad

**Provides: ½ Oil Unit, 1 Pulse Unit,
1 Seed Unit, ½ Quality Carb Unit**

60g brown rice (dry weight)
½ 400g can of mixed pulses, drained, OR beans of choice
  (see below)
50g small closed cap brown mushrooms OR shiitake
  mushrooms, sliced
1 medium red pepper, de-seeded and chopped
1 medium yellow pepper, de-seeded and chopped
5cm piece of cucumber, de-seeded and chopped
2 spring onions, chopped
1 small red eating apple, cored and chopped
1 seed mix portion (see page 40)
50g cooked sweetcorn kernels
½ a quantity of French Dressing (see recipe, page 156)
Mixed salad leaves

Cook the rice in boiling salted water until tender – between 30 and 45 minutes. Allow to cool slightly, then mix in all the rest of the ingredients, combine well and serve surrounded by mixed salad leaves.

○ Blackeyed or borlotti beans would go well.

Salade Nicoise

Provides: *1 Protein Unit, ½ Oil Unit,*
½ Quality Carb Unit

1 to 2 Little Gem lettuces
250g fresh tuna steak, lightly grilled OR 1 × 200g can tuna
    in olive oil, drained
4 small or 2 large tasty ripe tomatoes
50g cooked green beans, each cut in half
1 small red onion or 4 spring onions, sliced
5cm cucumber, diced
8 stoned black olives
6 anchovy fillets, drained and patted dry
½ a quantity of French Dressing (see recipe, page 156)

Cut the lettuce into segments and arrange in two serving bowls. Break the tuna into chunks and arrange on top. Roughly chop the tomatoes and add them with the beans, cucumber and onion to the dish. Arrange the olives and anchovies on top and drizzle the dressing over.

o   For the maintenance diet, hardboiled egg quarters and some cold cooked new potatoes can be added to this dish.

Orange and Rice Salad

Provides: *½ Oil Unit, 1 Seed Unit,*
1 Quality Carb Unit, ½ C-Fruit Unit

50g basmati and wild rice (dry weight)
1 orange
1 seed mix portion (see page 40)
50g fresh beansprouts
4 dried ready-to-eat apricots, chopped
1 dessertspoon light tahini
2 tablespoons salad oil blend (see page 34)

Sea salt
Black pepper
Flat-leaved parsley to garnish

Cook the rice in boiling lightly salted water until tender; drain if necessary. Segment the orange, retaining any juice that runs out, then combine the orange and seed mix with the rice, beansprouts and apricots. Beat the tahini into the oil blend, add the seasoning and the orange juice and beat again. Pour this dressing over the rice mixture and combine well. Serve garnished with flat-leaved parsley.

○ Add a teaspoon of ground cumin to the dressing blend, if you like.

Black Bean Salsa

Provides: *1 Pulse Unit, 1 Flame Unit, 1/2 Oil Unit*

200g cooked, drained black beans (see note below)
2 large tasty tomatoes, de-seeded and chopped (leave skin on)
1 red pepper, de-seeded and chopped
5cm cucumber, de-seeded and chopped
1 red chilli pepper, de-seeded and finely chopped
1 small red onion, chopped
2 tablespoons salad oil blend (see page 34)
1 tablespoon lime juice
Good handful fresh chopped coriander leaves
Sea salt
Black pepper

In a bowl, combine all the ingredients well, cover and chill for an hour or so before serving.

○ Red kidney beans or blackeyed beans can be used instead. Home cooked or canned, well-drained beans are both fine.

Panzanella

Provides: *½ Quality Carb Unit,*
1 Flame Unit, ½ Oil Unit

> 2 slices crusty good stoneground wholewheat bread
> 2 to 3 ripe tasty tomatoes, de-seeded and chopped
> 5cm piece cucumber, de-seeded and chopped
> 1 small red onion, thinly sliced
> 8 stoned black olives
> Dessertspoonful rinsed capers
> 1 good clove garlic, crushed
> 2 tablespoons tomato juice
> 2 tablespoons olive oil
> 1 tablespoon red wine vinegar
> Sea salt
> Black pepper
> Handful fresh basil leaves

Lightly toast the bread and break it into pieces. Put the bread, tomatoes, cucumber, onion, olives and capers into a serving bowl or two individual bowls. Mix together the garlic, tomato juice, olive oil, vinegar, salt and pepper and pour over the salad. Add the basil leaves and serve.

○ Flat-leaved parsley is a good alternative to basil, especially if serving with the sardines, as on Day Seven of the Omega Diet (page 114).

○ Capers can be omitted if you like, but they add a good piquancy to the salad.

Fruit, Nut and Pasta Salad

Provides: *1 Nut Unit, 1 Fruit-2 Unit,*
½ Oil Unit, ½ Quality Carb Unit

> 6 good quality dried ready-to-eat apricots, chopped
> Handful seedless red grapes, halved
> 1 tablespoon pine nuts

1 tablespoon roughly chopped pecan nuts
1 tablespoon roughly chopped walnuts
1 level tablespoon seed mix (see page 40)
75g broccoli florets, lightly steamed or boiled until just tender and
    drained
60g wholewheat pasta shapes (dry weight), boiled until tender
    and drained
½ quantity French Dressing (see recipe, page 156)
Mixed salad leaves

Combine all the ingredients except the salad leaves in a bowl and serve in individual dishes on the salad leaves.

Tabbouleh

Provides: ½ Oil Unit, 1 Quality Carb Unit

80g bulghar wheat (dry weight)
1 tub flat-leaved parsley, de-stalked and chopped
Good handful fresh mint, de-stalked and chopped
4 spring onions, chopped
2 good sized tasty ripe tomatoes, de-seeded and chopped
8cm piece cucumber, de-seeded and chopped
2 tablespoons salad oil blend (see page 34)
Juice of ½ lemon
Sea salt
Black pepper

Put the bulghar wheat in a bowl and pour over 200ml boiling water. Leave to stand until the water has been absorbed and the wheat is tender. If there is any excess liquid, drain it off thoroughly. Add all the remaining ingredients and serve the salad in shallow bowls.

Classic Waldorf Salad

Provides: *1 Nut Unit, 1 Fruit–2 Unit*

1 large red dessert apple
3 tablespoons roughly chopped walnuts
4 smallish tender sticks celery, chopped
2 tablespoons sultanas
3 tablespoons natural low-fat bio yogurt
1 tablespoon low-fat natural fromage frais
1 dessertspoon lemon juice
Pinch brown caster sugar
Sea salt
Black pepper
Some celery leaves

Core and chop the apple and place in a bowl with the celery, nuts and sultanas. In another bowl, combine the next six ingredients until you have a smooth dressing. Check for seasoning and pour on to the salad, combining well. Serve the salad garnished with the celery leaves.

Italian Three Bean Salad

Provides: *½ Oil Unit, 1 Pulse Unit*

150g cooked drained (or canned and drained) cannellini beans
150g small tender broad beans, cooked and drained
50g green beans, cooked until barely tender, drained and halved
100g canned red peppers, drained and thinly sliced
4 good quality artichoke hearts (from a can or jar), well drained
    and halved
1 small mild onion, thinly sliced
Small handful flat-leaved parsley, de-stalked and chopped
1 quantity of French Dressing (see recipe, page 156)

Combine all the ingredients lightly in a bowl and serve.

Main Meals

Rainbow Trout Fillets with Tapenade

Provides: *1 Protein Unit, ½ Oil Unit*

2 filleted (skin still on) rainbow trouts
12 good quality stoned black olives
4 anchovy fillets, drained and dried
1 good clove garlic, peeled
1 level tablespoon chopped parsley
2 tablespoons salad oil blend (see page 34)
Black pepper, and sea salt if needed

Heat the grill and when very hot put the filleted trouts, skin side up, to grill. Meanwhile, blend all the rest of the ingredients in an electric mill or with pestle and mortar until you have a thick paste-like sauce. Check for seasoning and add salt if needed. After a few minutes the trout will be cooked. Serve skin-side down with half the sauce on each.

Catalan Tuna with Tomato Sauce

**Provides: *1 Protein Unit, ½ Oil Unit,
1 Flame Unit***

2 tablespoons olive oil
2 fresh tuna steaks
1 medium onion, finely chopped
1 good clove garlic, crushed
1 medium red pepper, de-seeded and chopped
200g canned chopped tomatoes
1 level tablespoon sundried tomato paste
A little fish or vegetable stock
Juice of ¼ lemon
1 bay leaf
A few small closed cap mushrooms, sliced
Sea salt and black pepper

Heat the oil in a non-stick frying pan and when very hot, sear the tuna steaks on both sides (no more than 1 minute a side). Remove the steaks to a covered plate. Turn the heat down, add the onion and garlic to the pan with the red pepper and fry over a medium heat, stirring frequently, until soft and the onions are just turning golden – about 7 or 8 minutes.

Now add the rest of the ingredients, stir well and simmer for 20 minutes or until you have a good sauce. If things look too dry, add a little more stock and stir well. Put the tuna steaks back into the centre of the pan and simmer for a further few minutes until the tuna is just cooked.

○ Garnish with chopped black stoned olives and/or flat-leaved parsley if you like.

Spicy Stuffed Peppers

Provides: *1 Pulse Unit, 1 Flame Unit, ½ Oil Unit*

   1 tablespoon olive oil
   1 Spanish onion, finely chopped
   1 good clove garlic, crushed
   1 green chilli, de-seeded and chopped
   50g chestnut mushrooms, chopped
   1 large tomato, chopped
   200g brown or green canned lentils, drained weight
   1 dessertspoon sundried tomato paste
   50ml tomato juice or passata
   3 tablespoons Tabbouleh (see recipe, page 143) OR wholemeal
      breadcrumbs mixed with chopped mint
   Sea salt and black pepper
   2 orange or red peppers, halved and de-seeded

Heat the oil in a non-stick frying pan and fry the onion over a medium heat until soft, adding the garlic and chilli towards the end of cooking time. Add the mushrooms and stir everything well, then add the tomato, lentils, tomato paste and passata and simmer for 5 to 10 minutes.

Combine the mixture with the Tabbouleh (or breadcrumbs and mint), a little salt and pepper.

Pile the mixture into the pepper halves and put them in a shallow ovenproof dish with a few tablespoons of water in the bottom. Put into an oven at 200°C and bake for an hour or until tender. You may need to put small pieces of foil over the stuffing mixture if it look as if it is drying out or going too brown.

Chickpea, Spinach and Aubergine Harissa

Provides: ½ Oil Unit, 1 Green Unit, 1 Pulse Unit

1 aubergine
1½ tablespoons olive oil
1 medium onion, finely chopped
1 tablespoon harissa paste
200g canned chopped tomatoes
1 × 400g can chickpeas in water, drained and rinsed
1 bag leaf spinach
Sea salt, if necessary

Cut the aubergine into slices and then halve the slices. Toss in half the olive oil and arrange on a baking tray, then bake in a 210°C oven for 30 minutes, turning once, until they are golden and cooked through. Meanwhile, heat the rest of the oil in a non-stick frying pan and fry the onions over a medium heat, stirring frequently, until they are soft and just turning golden. Add two-thirds of the harissa and stir for a minute, then add the aubergine, tomatoes and chickpeas, cover and simmer for 20 to 30 minutes.

Meanwhile, wash the spinach and wilt it in a saucepan with no extra water until just reduced but not overcooked.

To serve, add the remaining harissa to the chickpea mixture and stir for a minute. Add the spinach and stir again. Check seasoning, adding a little sea salt if necessary, and serve.

Mexican Chilli

Provides: *½ Oil Unit, 1 Flame Unit,*
1 Pulse Unit, ½ Calcium Unit

200g soya mince
2 tablespoons olive oil
1 large onion, finely chopped
1 fresh red chilli and 1 green chilli, chopped (see note below)
200g can chopped tomatoes
200g can red kidney beans OR blackeyed beans,
    drained and rinsed
Teaspoon vegetable stock powder
Sea salt
Black pepper
Handful fresh coriander leaves
150ml low-fat bio yogurt

Reconstitute the soya mince according to pack instructions. Heat the oil in a non-stick frying pan and fry the onion over a medium heat until it is soft and just turning golden. Add the chilli and stir again, then add the mince, turn the heat up a little and stir for a few minutes to colour it.

Add the tomatoes, beans, stock powder and seasoning and bring to simmer, adding a little water if necessary. Simmer for 30 minutes until you have a good sauce, then check seasoning and serve garnished with fresh coriander and yogurt.

○ You can use lean minced beef in this recipe if you are on a meat protein day.
○ You may like to use more chilli, or make the dish hotter by including the chilli seeds. If the chillies you have bought are particularly mild, you can add a teaspoon or so of dried chilli powder or dried crushed chillies to make the dish hotter.

Falafel Patties

Provides: *1 Pulse Unit*

1 × 400g can cooked chickpeas, drained and rinsed
1 small to medium onion, very finely chopped
1 canned red pepper, drained and finely chopped
1 clove garlic, crushed
1 tablespoon mixed chopped parsley, coriander and mint
    (see note below)
½ teaspoon each freshly ground coriander and cumin
White of an egg, beaten
Sea salt
Black pepper
A little wholemeal, chickpea or soya flour
1 teaspoon olive oil

Mash the chickpeas well with a fork in a bowl (or use a blender). Add the onion, pepper, garlic, herbs, spices, egg white and seasoning and mix well, then form into four patties. Coat these in the flour. Heat a griddle or good quality nonstick frying pan and brush with the oil. When the pan or griddle is medium hot, cook the patties for a few minutes, turning once, until they are golden on each side. Serve immediately.

o   You can use one or all of these. If you are going to pick one, my own preference is coriander.

Mushroom and Lentil Hotpot

Provides: *1 Pulse Unit, ¼ Oil Unit*

100ml dark beer or red wine
1 tablespoon Worcestershire or soya sauce
200ml vegetable stock
100g brown or Puy lentils
1 medium onion, chopped
1 good clove garlic, crushed
1 tablespoon olive oil
400g large dark-gilled mushrooms, sliced
1 sprig fresh oregano
1 bay leaf
2 sprigs fresh thyme
1 tablespoon fresh chopped parsley
Black pepper
Little sea salt, if necessary

Put the beer, Worcestershire sauce and stock into a fairly large saucepan, add the lentils and simmer for 30 minutes or until tender. Meanwhile, heat the oil in a nonstick frying pan and fry the onion and garlic for a few minutes until soft, then add the mushrooms and herbs and stir for a minute. Set the pan off the heat if the lentils aren't cooked yet; otherwise, tip the mushroom and onion mixture into the pan of lentils, stir well, add black pepper, cover and simmer for 15 minutes or until the mushrooms are cooked but not too mushy. Check seasoning, salt if necessary and serve.

○ Add a teaspoon of fresh chopped chilli or ginger to this dish if you like.
○ A spoonful of low-fat bio yogurt or fromage frais stirred in before serving is nice.

Lemon Lamb Kebabs with Tzatziki

Provides: *½ Oil Unit, 1 Protein Unit, 1 Quality Carb Unit, ½ Calcium Unit*

> 300g or so of lean lamb (leg or neck fillet)
> ½ juicy lemon
> 2 tablespoons olive oil
> 2 large cloves garlic, crushed
> Teaspoon fresh chopped rosemary
> Black pepper
> Sea salt
> 1 large orange pepper, de-seeded and cut into squares
> 1 medium red onion, peeled and cut into squares
> 2 wholewheat pittas
> 1 small tub half-fat Greek yogurt
> Teaspoon white wine vinegar
> 5cm piece cucumber

Cut the lamb into bite-sized cubes and put in a shallow dish. Pour over the oil, the juice from the lemon, add two-thirds of the garlic, the seasoning and rosemary, combine well with your hands, cover and allow to marinate for at least an hour. When ready to cook, heat the grill to high, thread the lamb pieces alternately on to kebab sticks with the red onion and orange pepper, brush with the marinade, and grill for about 8 minutes, turning once or twice and basting each time.

Meanwhile, mix the yogurt with the vinegar and the rest of the garlic. Halve, de-seed and chop the cucumber and then squeeze much of the moisture out using strong kitchen paper, and add the cucumber to the yogurt. Stir well and season.

When the kebabs are ready, serve with the pittas and tzatziki plus plenty of mixed salad leaves.

o   This also works well with lean pork fillet.

Chicken and Pasta Casserole

*Provides: ½ Oil Unit, 1 Protein Unit,
1 Flame Unit, ½ Quality Carb Unit*

2 tablespoons olive oil
4 boned and skinned chicken thighs
1 onion, chopped
1 large leek, washed and sliced
3 medium carrots, peeled and chopped
150ml chicken stock
100ml passata
1 level tablespoon sundried tomato paste
Sea salt
Black pepper
Few sprigs fresh, or 1 heaped teaspoon dried, thyme
60g wholewheat pasta spirals

Preheat the oven to 150°C. Heat the oil in a flameproof casserole and brown the chicken pieces on all sides; remove with a slotted spoon. Now add the onion and leek to the casserole and sauté over a medium heat until soft, stirring frequently. Now add all the remaining ingredients to the casserole, stir, cover and cook in the oven for one hour or until the chicken, vegetables and pasta are tender. Check seasoning and serve.

Pork and Cashews with Noodles

Provides: ½ Oil Unit,
1 Protein Unit, 1 Nut Unit,
1 Seed Unit, 1 Green Unit,
1 Flame Unit, ½ Quality Carb Unit

60g wholewheat egg thread noodles
1½ tablespoons olive oil
250g pork fillet, sliced
1 red pepper, de-seeded and thinly sliced
100g shredded savoy cabbage
100g pak choi
1 dessertspoon sesame oil
1 tablespoon soya sauce
Piece ginger, peeled and finely chopped
1 clove garlic, finely chopped
1 red chilli, de-seeded and finely chopped
1 tablespoon hoisin sauce
Little vegetable stock
40g unsalted fresh cashew nuts or almonds
20g seed mix (see page 40)

Cook the noodles in boiling water for a few minutes or as instructed on pack, until just tender; drain and reserve. Heat the oil in a wok or large non-stick frying pan and stir-fry the pork and red pepper over a high heat until the pork is golden (about 3 minutes). Add the cabbage and pak choi with the sesame oil, and stir-fry for a few more minutes, then add the soya sauce, ginger, garlic and chilli and stir for a minute. Add the hoisin sauce, a little stock as necessary, and the nuts and stir for another minute. Before serving stir in the noodles and seeds to warm through. Serve immediately.

○ A similar stir-fry can be made substituting chicken and almonds for the pork and cashews. Or you can swap the Protein Unit for a Pulse Unit by using tofu chunks instead of the meat. (See recipe for Marinated Tofu, page 157)

Mediterranean Meatballs in a Rich Sauce

**Provides: ½ Oil Unit, 1 Protein Unit,
1 Flame Unit**

250g extra-lean beef, minced
2 tablespoons stale wholewheat breadcrumbs
1 medium onion, very finely chopped
Handful fresh flat-leaved parsley, chopped
Half a teaspoon ground cumin seed
1 egg white, beaten
Sea salt
Black pepper
2 tablespoons olive oil
1 small red pepper, de-seeded and finely chopped
1 clove garlic, crushed
200g chopped tomatoes with Mediterranean herbs
100ml passata
Pinch brown caster sugar
1 dessertspoon sundried tomato paste
4 stoned black olives, halved

In a bowl, combine the meat, crumbs, onion, parsley, cumin and egg white with some seasoning. Form into 10 small balls. Heat half the oil in a lidded non-stick frying pan or flameproof casserole and brown the meatballs over a medium high heat for a few minutes, turning several times. Remove with slotted spoon, add rest of oil and sauté the red pepper for a few minutes, stirring frequently and adding the garlic towards the end of this process. Then add the rest of the ingredients, stir well, return the meatballs to the pan, cover and allow to simmer for 20 to 30 minutes or until you have a rich sauce. Check seasoning and serve.

○ Serve with a Quality Carb Unit such as wholewheat spaghetti, brown rice or bulghar wheat.

Miscellaneous

Dried Fruit Breakfast Compote

Provides: *1 Fruit-2 Unit*

> 50g dried apricots
> 25g dried stoned prunes
> 25g dried figs
> 25g dried pears
> 100ml orange juice
> Pinch ground ginger
> Pinch ground cinnamon
> Water

Soak the fruits for a few hours or overnight in the orange juice with the spices and a dash of water added as necessary to cover. Simmer the fruit and juice mixture in a small saucepan for 15 to 20 minutes, adding a little extra water if necessary to barely cover. Serve warm or cold.

○ The compote can be transferred to an airtight container and kept in the fridge for a few days as necessary.

Apricot and Apple Milkshake

Provides: *1 Fruit-2 Unit, 1 Calcium Unit*

2 fresh, juicy eating apples
25g dried apricots, chopped and soaked for an hour or two in a
    little water or orange juice
350ml skimmed milk or soya milk
2 teaspoons runny honey
Pinch of ground cinnamon

Peel, core and chop the apples and process them in a blender. Add the apricots, half the milk, honey and cinnamon to the blender and process until you have a smooth pureé, then add the rest of the milk and blend again. Chill and serve.

- If you like, use a peach, pear or nectarine instead of the apple.
- To add half a Pulse Unit to this shake, blend in 100g of silken tofu with the first half of the milk.
- For a complete Pulse Unit, blend in 200g silken tofu with the fruit and add soya milk or water to give a good shake consistency.

French Dressing

Provides: *The complete recipe makes approximately four portions, and therefore contains ½ Oil Unit per portion, but amounts used in the recipes vary.*

4 tablespoons salad oil blend (see page 34)
1 tablespoon red or white wine vinegar
½ level teaspoon brown caster sugar
½ level teaspoon wholegrain French mustard
Sea salt
Black pepper

Shake together all ingredients in a screw-top jar. Check seasoning. This dressing will keep indefinitely in the fridge.

○ Add crushed garlic, or chopped fresh herbs, or chillies for a change – in which case the dressing should be consumed within days.

Marinated Tofu

Provides: *1 Pulse Unit, ¼ Oil Unit*

1 × 250g pack firm unsmoked tofu
50ml soya sauce
1 tablespoon salad oil blend (see page 34)
Dash of red wine
Dash of water
1 large clove garlic, very well crushed
2cm piece fresh ginger, peeled and finely chopped
One or two drops of hot chilli sauce

Slice or cut the tofu into cubes, depending upon what the recipe you're using calls for, and place in a small bowl or container. In another bowl, mix together all the marinade ingredients thoroughly, then pour over the tofu, stirring well. Cover and leave to marinate for an hour or two. The marinade should cover the tofu, but if it doesn't, stir from time to time. The leftover marinade can be kept for a week or so and re-used for more tofu, or in stir-fries, etc.

○ For using Marinated Tofu, see ideas on pages 126–8.

CHAPTER 8

Omega Plus – the Lifelong Solution

Ω

Weight maintenance, as most of us are no doubt all too aware, is harder than weight loss. At least, this is the theory based on most people's experience.

It doesn't have to be that way. If you have lost weight by eating a completely healthy and varied diet, then staying slim by persisting with that diet (albeit MORE of it, calorie-wise) isn't a difficult task at all.

The Omega Plus system simply builds on what has gone before. If you took the leap of faith involved in eating the Omega Units way to lose weight, and are enjoying the body and health benefits it brings, then you will be happy to continue eating in a similar way. There are no more major changes involved – the Omega Plus system adds more variety and more calories to your diet but that is all. It is the natural way to stay slim and healthy.

The Omega Plus system

As regards your maintenance plan, all you need to do is three things:

1. *Add a wider range of foods* to those allowed within the original 12 units, to give you more choice.
2. *Add extra calories* to your mainentance diet by adding on extra quantity of the units.
3. *Add a range of extra treats* to your diet.

A wider range of choices within the units

First, we add extra foods to some of the units, to provide you with more choice and variety on your maintenance diet.

Unit One – Protein Unit

The complete list of choices for this unit appears on page 33 in Chapter 2. To this list you can now ADD:

Ω *Eggs* A portion of eggs is 2 to 3 medium eggs, cooked any way you want (but if frying, use oil from your Oil Unit). Eggs contain iron, B vitamins including folate, vitamins A, D and E. They also contain 6g of fat per average egg, of which about 2g is saturated. They're high in cholesterol, but up to two egg meals a week will be fine. Have your omega-3 fish oil capsule with your egg meal.

Ω *Cheese* Hard cheeses such as Cheddar, blue cheeses such as Stilton, St Agur, blue brie, and cream cheeses such as mascarpone are very high in fat and saturated fat and, except as a very occasional item, are best avoided. However, you can include other cheeses on your Omega Plus plan in up to two meals a week, which will also boost your calcium intake.

Choose from goat's cheese, halloumi, feta, mozzarella or any other cheese labelled as containing not more than 22g of total fat per 100g weight.

A portion of these cheeses is around 50g.

You can also have cottage cheese, low-fat soft cheese and fromage frais – a portion of these is around 75 to 100g.

Have your omega-3 fish oil capsules with your cheese meal.

NOTE: As these join unit one, your Protein Unit, you shouldn't eat them in total more than twice a week – that is, two egg meals or two cheese meals or one egg meal plus one cheese meal. This then will still leave room for your other protein foods (such as fish, poultry, meat or Quorn) and you will still be getting a wide variety of protein foods in your diet. And you shouldn't eat egg or cheese meals instead of your Pulse Unit, by the way.

Unit Two – Oil Unit

The complete list of choices for your Oil Unit appears on page 34 in Chapter 2.

An alternative salad blend (particularly useful if you aren't keen on the taste of walnut oil) is to use 50% soya oil, 40% extra virgin olive oil and 10% linseed oil. Another is to use 50% rapeseed oil, 40% groundnut oil and 10% linseed oil.

You can buy linseed oil from health food shops. It should be stored in the shop in a cool place and be fresh – it has a short shelf life. Treat it like gold dust at home, storing in the fridge in an opaque container, and use it up within a few weeks. Some linseed oil tastes better than others. It is important in these salad mixes to add the linseed oil as it is so high in omega-3s and puts back what you have lost by omitting the walnut oil.

NOTE: Oils are – or should be – genuine health foods and you should treat them with respect. Get as much of your oil as you can uncooked, and buy the best quality oil you can, always – that is, unrefined, cold-pressed, extra virgin, organic and so on. Refined commercial oils have little goodness left in them. Genuine oils are full of healthy micronutrients. If possible, buy your oil in a specialist shop (or, these days, mail order or on the Internet). Store oils carefully and use them up within weeks.

Unit Three – Nut Unit

The unit three nut mix recipe appears on page 36 in Chapter 2.

Some alternative nuts that you can eat from time to time on the Omega Plus plan are: almonds, brazils, pecans, macadamias.

A portion of nuts is about 20g shelled weight.

Don't forget to buy your nuts really fresh (preferably with shells still on), store them in an airtight container in a cool place and eat them within weeks. Whole nuts will keep better than chopped or broken nuts so if you do buy them shelled, don't buy nut pieces, which probably will contain little of the original oils.

Unit Four – Seed Unit

The unit four seed mix recipe appears on page 40 in Chapter 2.

On your Omega Plus plan, other seeds can be added to the diet as you like. Extra linseeds can be sprinkled on to salads or your breakfast cereal; pine nuts can be used in salads and dressings; poppy and sesame seeds can be used similarly.

You just need to remember that only linseeds and pumpkin seeds contain good amounts of the vital omega-3 fatty acids, so don't eat other seeds at the expense of these.

Units Five and Six – C-Fruit and Fruit-2 Units

The complete unit five and six lists appears on pages 58–9 in Chapter 3.

If you find any other fruits at all that you would like to add to your diet, treat them as Fruit-2 choices. One obvious example here is avocados (fruits, not vegetables!). They weren't on the slimming diet as they are very high in fat, but on a maintenance plan they are excellent food – high in mono-unsaturates, vitamin B6 and vitamin E, as well as being a good source of both types of fibre and potassium.

Units Seven and Eight – Green and Flame Units

The complete unit seven and eight lists appear on pages 59–60 in Chapter 3.

If you find any other vegetables that you would like to add to your diet and which don't appear on the lists, do so from time to time, but if the edible parts aren't green or flame-coloured, don't eat them at the expense of the items on the unit seven and eight lists, but try to eat them in addition. (By the way, don't forget that a long list of vegetables also appears on the 'unlimited' list on page 105 – check the list out to see if your other chosen veggies appear on it. Onions of all kinds, for example, are unlimited.)

Most vegetables contain very few calories and are unlikely to make you put on weight! Most vegetables, even those not coloured green or flame, or on the unlimited list, will have valuable trace elements, phytochemicals and so on, to improve your overall diet.

Unit Nine – Pulse Unit

The complete list of pulses appears on page 73 in Chapter 4. If any pulse that you want to eat doesn't appear on the list, by all means add it. All pulses are good.

Unit Ten – Quality Carb Unit

The complete list of Omega carbohydrates appears on page 84 in Chapter 5. This list is quite comprehensive, but you may want to add the occasional baked potato, or 'old' potato in its many guises, to your diet. That is fine. An average baking potato is a portion.

Units Eleven and Twelve – Calcium and Water Units

The complete list of items in these units appears on pages 89 and 95 in Chapter 5. These units contain the same choices on the Omega Plus plan.

Adding extra calories

Once you are down to the weight you want to be, you need to eat more calories to maintain your new weight. For most people, this will represent around 500 extra calories or so a day or about a third more calories – but of course this varies. You will soon find out how much extra you can eat without beginning to put weight on again. If you carry on with the Omega principles, you won't find hunger a problem and so you shouldn't be tempted to eat too many calories.

An important Omega principle to remember is that you eat for health, nutrition and pleasure. You don't eat for greed!

There is one simple way to add extra calories, and that is to add extra units to your diet.

While you were slimming, you had 12 units a day. On the Omega Plus system, you simply double up some of the units until you are eating enough calories to maintain your weight.

The first one to start with is the Quality Carb Unit. On the Omega slimming diet, we limited this unit, but for long-term health, larger portions of carbohydrates are a good idea. So getting TWO Quality Carb Units instead of one will add around 180 to 200 calories a day to your diet. Simply check through the Quality Carb Unit list on page 84 and choose two items rather than one (such as 6 slices of bread rather than 3, or one 60g portion pasta plus one 3-slice portion of bread, or one sweet potato plus one 60g portion brown rice. The choice of combination is up to you).

The second is the Calcium Unit. You can happily eat TWO Calcium units a day, which will add about 100 calories.

Thirdly, consider getting two Pulse Units a day, at least occasionally, as these are so very good for you. Alternatively, you could double your Nut or Seed Units to provide extra essential fats in your diet. So aim to get an extra Pulse, Nut or Seed Unit every day.

When doubling any unit, you can either simply double the quantity of the portion you would normally have, or get the extra unit at a different time of day (the preferred solution).

These measures will increase your day's calorie intake by about 30%. If you then take on board some of the extra treats (see next paragraph) you will find your maintenance diet plan is 'full up' with no great change in your new eating habits at all.

Add a range of extra treats to your diet

Alcohol, chocolate, cakes, cappuccino, butter – if one or more of these are diet items that you still miss despite your changed tastebuds after weeks on the Omega Diet, don't feel too deprived. You needn't say goodbye to any of them on the Omega Plus plan.

If you choose wisely, are in good health and don't go overboard on quantity, all five can be included in your maintenance diet. Let's look at each of the five in turn.

Alcohol All alcohol – but particularly red wine and dark beers – contains anti-oxidant compounds called flavonoids which are linked with reduced risk of heart disease, particularly in people of middle age and over if intake is moderate. The alcohol itself also protects, by reducing the 'stickiness' of the blood and increasing levels of HDL cholesterol. The professional overview on alcohol is that moderate drinkers appear to live longer and have less heart disease than non-drinkers.

So if you want a glass of wine or beer with your evening meal, and you can spare the calories, then go ahead. If, however, you can't drink one or two glasses without wanting six or seven – it's perhaps better to avoid alcohol altogether. The good news is that red grape juice also contains the important flavonoids, so it's almost as good for the heart! Organic wine or beer will be less likely to give you a headache because it is made without the myriad of additives that normal alcoholic drinks are made with, so choose those if possible.

Chocolate Good quality dark chocolate also contains good amounts of anti-oxidants, as well as magnesium and iron. It can dilate the arteries and help the flow of blood, thus reducing the risk of heart attacks, American research confirms. So, again, if you can spare the calories, have a little chocolate every day. However, make sure that it is rich in cocoa solids (70% is ideal), and preferably organic.

Cakes There is cake – and cake. What you are allowed on the Omega Plus plan is an occasional slice of good quality, nutrient-rich cake. That means a cake made with good, wholesome ingredients such as organic eggs, wholemeal flour, dried fruits and so on. You need to bake it yourself, or buy it from a known local supplier, fresh. With such a cake, you will be getting iron, fibre, B vitamins, magnesium and many other nutrients, so you don't need to feel guilty. We discuss other types of cake later!

Cappuccino A cup of cappuccino – or, indeed, filtered or instant or espresso coffee – is quite definitely not the health hazard that some people will have you believe. It is true that if you overindulge in strong coffee you may find side-effects such as hyperactivity brought on by the caffeine; it is also true that you shouldn't drink coffee with a meal, as it may hinder absorption of minerals such as calcium and iron; and it is true that it can't count towards your day's fluid intake as it acts as a diuretic. And for women prone to breast pain/tenderness, it may be wise to avoid caffeine-rich drinks.

But otherwise the right kind of coffee between meals once or even twice a day will do you no harm and, research shows, helps to keep you alert and your concentration levels up.

The reason that cappuccino, filtered, instant and espresso coffees are the best is that they contain low levels of cafestol and kahweol, micro chemicals found in greatest concentration in cafetiere-brewed, percolated and Turkish coffee. These chemicals have been shown to raise the level of dangerous blood fats, including cholesterols and triglycerides.

Coffee, by the way, may dilate the airways and help to relieve asthma, can act as a laxative and helps to improve memory. As with most things that we eat or drink, moderation with coffee is definitely the key, but if the odd cup helps you to feel good about the world, then don't think it is going to do you untold harm.

NOTE: Don't count any milk you may use in coffee towards your day's Calcium Unit, as the chemicals in coffee may prevent its absorption.

Butter High in saturated fat, but, at least, a natural product, butter adds its own unique flavour to foods and you should use small amounts in your cooking occasionally without feeling guilty. For example, a knob added to your oil when sautéing or for roasting will impart flavour, or it can be added to scrambled eggs. If you avoid high-fat commercial produce (see below) then a little bit of butter won't do you any harm. If you can afford the calories, allow yourself about 35g a week (7 teaspoons) of butter, in addition to your Oil Units.

NOTE: You will probably notice that I talk a lot about 'good quality' in food. When you choose 'treat' items, it is important to buy the best quality that you can, whether it is alcohol or coffee, butter or chocolate, or cake ingredients. Try to eat wholesome, unadulterated, best-quality foods. In general, these will taste better, be more satisfying and do you more good. (See 'The importance of organic', opposite.)

Foods to avoid, long-term

Had you noticed that throughout this book I have hardly talked at all about what foods you shouldn't eat? That is because I have been so busy telling you all about the gorgeous array of fine foods you CAN eat that I just haven't had the occasion to do so.

Here seems as good a place as any to mention a few guidelines on foods to avoid. As a general rule, anything that isn't mentioned within the 14-day Omega Diet (plus unlimiteds), or the Freeform Diet, or the Omega Plus plan, is something you should avoid. This includes most foods which you will see in the supermarket that are high in saturated fat and particularly trans fats (see Chapter 2); or that combine fat and sugar together in high amounts (such as commercial cakes, biscuits, desserts, pastries, cheap chocolate); or that have long lists of additives (packet cakes, sweets, soups, food mixes, soft drinks and plenty more); or that are high in salt (packet mixes, canned soups, some ready meals, a variety of canned foods, stock cubes, sauces and plenty more); and foods which have been robbed of most of their wholesomeness by the manufacturing process (most of the items already mentioned in this paragraph as well as white bread and white pasta).

Your body doesn't need these foods, and your tastebuds don't need these foods, so don't buy them. And this seems a good point to bring in a few more words about organic food . . .

The importance of organic

I have urged you to buy specific organic produce several times within this book, and here I will reinforce the message with a more general plea.

In choosing the Omega Diet you have chosen a healthy, natural way to eat. It therefore makes sense to take it one step further and choose to eat organically as much as you possibly can. Why spoil a healthy diet with pesticides, hormones, additives, possibly genetically modified ingredients and so on, when you can buy your food without any worry about them containing these things, and other undesirables?

One important factor is the 'cumulative effect'. Because you have increased the amount of fruits, vegetables, salads and wholegrains that you eat, you will be ingesting more pesticides and other 'undesirables' than on a typical Western diet, which contains these items in much smaller amounts. The British Government tests samples of our farmed produce regularly and decrees that most of the tested foods contain residues that are well within safety limits for human consumption. But this really doesn't take account of the add-on effect. It is better to be safe . . .

Also, organic food does taste better, as proved by a recent test in Britain, and it tends to contain higher amounts of vitamins, minerals and phytochemicals. If you have a garden, I strongly urge you to start growing a few items of your own – the cheapest way to have organic food. Even on a patio you can grow fresh herbs, salad leaves, new potatoes, tomatoes and so on. Otherwise, you could visit farm shops where costs are lower, and perhaps split food packs with neighbours, or freeze any surplus.

If you can only buy some organic foods, make it leafy greens, especially lettuce. You can peel a potato or apple and remove residues, but not a cabbage or a Cos! (Having said that, much of the vitamin goodness of fruit and vegetables that you might peel does lie directly under the skin, so if you peel you will not only be throwing away possible residues, but also good nutrients.)

Carrots are also well worth buying organic as residues tend to be higher in these than in most other vegetables. Otherwise, remove the top 2cm and peel well.

Also buy organic lemons and limes if you are going to use the peel.

Organic fish, meat and poultry usually tastes infinitely superior and as on the Omega Diet you eat everything but fish in smaller quantities, perhaps, than you have been used to, you won't have to spend much more money.

Lastly, think about buying organic dried fruits, nuts, seeds and pulses. Dried fruits, in particular, may contain high levels of preservatives if not organic.

Even if you can't manage to buy everything organic, the Omega Diet is still more natural and lower in many artificial additives than the average consumer diet.

Eating out and entertaining

If you have embraced the Omega way of eating with enthusiasm, it won't be hard for you to seek out restaurants and other eating places where the food that is served is the kind of food that fits in with the Omega pattern. It is worthwhile doing some legwork and homework on which places these are, until you have built up a selection that will fulfil all your needs.

Even when you find yourself stuck, for social or work reasons, in an eating place which serves only additive-rich, highly refined food swimming in saturated fat, there are still some measures you can take to make the menu a bit more user-friendly for yourself.

Choose a starter based on fruit, salad or light vegetable soup if there are any; if not, say no and eat a piece of wholemeal bread instead (if there is any!). Plainly cooked main courses are the best bet – fish or poultry with vegetables, or a rice or pasta dish.

If the menu doesn't show what you want, it is always worth asking. (For instance, you can ask for a dish to be de-sauced.)

If you are a regular airline traveller you will know that some lines serve much better food than others; this must be an important consideration when booking your flight! I have found that if you ask for a vegan meal you may get something of more wholesome quality than otherwise. If you only travel on a plane once a year, packing your own sandwich for the flight is probably the sensible solution.

Holidaying or eating abroad, you should be able to find plenty of good things to eat. Almost any country I can think of will serve decent, good quality food at good prices, especially if you avoid eating in your hotel dining room. Local cafés with local produce should do you proud.

And at home, don't think that because you are entertaining you suddenly have to stop eating the Omega way and start serving food enriched with lashings of cream, full-fat cheese, sugar, salt and so on. Serve up what you like and your guests will like it too – unless you are a particularly bad cook! Cooking is a joy, and if you have spent years living on fast food, takeaways or ready meals for one or two, now is the time to practise your culinary skills. It is never too late to learn.

Special needs

If you are pregnant, or thinking of becoming pregnant, are ill, or convalescing, or have any medical condition in which diet is a factor, please do see your doctor and discuss the Omega Diet with him before beginning it. It is a healthy way to eat but it can't cover every eventuality and you may have special needs – you may be allergic to one or more of the foods mentioned, for instance. And alcohol, allowed on the Omega Plus Diet, may affect your chances of becoming pregnant and may even affect the pregnancy itself.

Very young children shouldn't follow the Omega Diet, as it may be too high in fibre and too 'bulky' for them. It also contains nuts, which children under five shouldn't eat.

Supplements

Apart from the omega-3 fish oil supplement, no other supplements are truly necessary on the Omega Diet or the Omega Plus plan, again, unless you have special needs. For example, when pregnant you should take folate supplements.

In general, supplements, especially vitamin and mineral supplements, don't work as well as the 'real thing', as part of food. They are less easily absorbed by the body, may cause imbalances, and may even cause more ills than they may cure.

The Omega Diet is especially rich in vitamin C, vitamin E, B vitamins, all the major minerals and essential fatty acids, and taking a supplement other than the omega-3 fish oil supplement on non-oily-fish days is unlikely to achieve anything.

The 13th Unit

There is one extra which you should add to your Omega Diet, right from the start and for the rest of your life. It is so important that I call it the 13th Omega Unit.

It is exercise.

Keeping active on a regular daily basis is the key that is missing in the lives of many overweight and unfit people. Exercise has so very many benefits that if you don't take any, you really are missing out on optimum health, however good your diet may be.

Exercise works synergistically with food to keep you well.

So please, every day, or at least 4 to 5 days a week, do some exercise for about 30 minutes. Walking is the best choice for most people as it is relatively easy, costs nothing and needs no special equipment.

Get out and walk at a pace that has you feeling very slightly 'puffed out', but not over-exerted. As the days go by, you will get fitter and you will walk faster to achieve the same effect.

Later you might try cycling or swimming. If you like to exercise indoors, you could try an exercise bike or rower or a skiing machine.

Exercise gets your heart fit and burns off calories. It improves quality of sleep and concentration, aids relaxation, and plenty more. So think of exercise as a necessary part of the total Omega system – and do it!

In conclusion

I hope that you have learned plenty of new and useful facts from this book and that it has inspired you to think carefully about what you put into your mouth, and why.

As I said at the start, it isn't always easy to make food changes or to stick with a way of eating that isn't exactly the normal way in our fast-food-dominated society. But it WILL get easier.

As more and more people demand better and better food, then the shops and food outlets will begin to try to provide it (indeed, they are beginning now), the farming industry will have to change, and the Omega way of eating will, eventually, become the norm.

Remember, it is only a few years ago that vegetarians, for example, were hard pushed to find any choices on restaurant menus. Now they are spoilt for choice. Things can change, and things do change.

The sellers are, ultimately, led by you, the buyer, however much it may seem to the contrary. You just need to know what you want, and keep demanding it.

The future is Omega. Be sure of it.

Do You Need To Lose Weight?

Measure your height without shoes, weight without outer clothes and waist circumference and then check out the two charts below.

The first assesses your health risk by your weight and height and is based on the Body Mass Index system, which is internationally recognised as an accurate measurement system. Using a ruler, simply find the point at which your height line (vertical) meets your weight line (horizontal). Then read off the weight diagnosis. For example, if you are 68ins tall and weigh 13½ stone (189lb), your point lies almost exactly in the centre of the 'overweight' section, c.

The Body Mass Index Chart

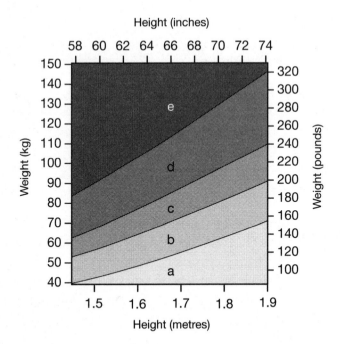

What the readings mean

The guidelines for interpreting your results are as follows:

a – Underweight (BMI 20 or below) You do not need to lose any more weight and being underweight may cause health problems, especially long term.

b – Normal weight (BMI 20–25) This is an acceptable weight range and for your health's sake you don't need to lose any weight (or gain any weight). However if your 'point' is at or near the next band up, check out the Ashwell Shape Chart below for further instructions.

c – Overweight (BMI 25–30) Within this band, your weight may cause health problems, especially long-term, and this is increasingly likely the further to the right of the chart your 'point' falls. You should lose some weight, especially if your waist circumference is large (see Ashwell Shape Chart below).

d – Very overweight (BMI 30–40) You are clinically obese and there is a real risk of current and future weight-related health problems and reduced lifespan. You should lose weight until your body mass index falls into the band below, and, long-term, aim to get your weight into the upper end of the 'normal' category.

e – Extremely overweight (BMI over 40) Weights in this range are classed as 'morbidly obese' which means you have a high likelihood of weight-related health problems including CHD, and early death.

The Ashwell Shape Chart

Research shows that if you tend to carry fat around your middle, rather than your hips or thighs, for instance, you are at higher risk of heart disease, diabetes and other health problems. Margaret Ashwell, ex-scientific director of the British Nutrition Foundation, devised the chart overleaf to show just how much (or how little) of a risk your own shape presents.

Using the same process as on the chart above, find your 'point' on the chart and read off the health risk assessment for your own waistline. This is particularly useful if you are a 'borderline' case on the weight chart. For example, if your 'point' was at the upper end of 'normal' on the weight chart but your waistline shows 'OK', then you needn't worry; your weight is almost certainly fine. But if it shows 'take care', then you need to lose some weight and do more exercise to get your waist measurement down into the 'OK' range.

Similarly, your weight chart results may have been 'overweight' but your shape chart may say 'OK'. This means your surplus weight is distributed in your lower body (and/or chest) and poses much less of a health risk. Losing weight will then be cosmetic rather than a health necessity.

If you come into the 'overweight', 'very overweight' or 'extremely overweight' category on the weight chart AND into either the 'take care' or 'at risk' category on the shape chart, then it is certain that you do, indeed, need to lose weight.

The Ashwell Shape Chart

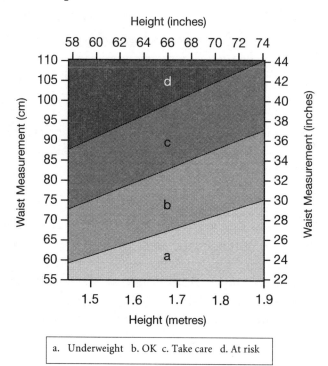

a. Underweight   b. OK   c. Take care   d. At risk

Nutritional Information

Macronutrient content of the Omega slimming diet

(14-day diet and Freeform)
(All figures approximate only as there are variables within the diet and portion sizes will vary)

Nutrient	% of total calories
Protein	20%
Carbohydrate	50%
Total fat	30%

Fat analysis	% of total calories
Saturated fats	4%
Mono-unsaturated fats	15%
Polyunsaturated omega-6 fats	7%*
Polyunsaturated omega-3 fats	4%*
(Total polyunsaturates	11%*)

(*Based on using the olive oil/rapeseed oil blend as Oil Unit. If salad blend is used as preferred oil, omega-6 content and total polyunsaturated fat content will be slightly higher, and omega-3 content slightly lower. If plain olive oil is used as preferred oil, total mono-unsaturated fat content will be slightly higher, and both omega-6 content and omega-3 content slightly lower.)

Maintenance diet (Omega Plus)

Proportions of nutrients will remain approximately the same but with greater chance for variables.

APPENDIX 3

Addresses

Fish oil capsules: Unpolluted fish oil capsules can be obtained from Higher Nature, who do a mail order service. Tel: 01435 882880.

Organic foods: Further information can be obtained from:
The Soil Association, 96 Colston Road, Bristol, BS1 5BB,
tel: 0117 929 0661. Send a SAE for list of organic suppliers in your area, or ring for other advice.
The Organic Directory 2000/2001. This book is co-published at £7.95 by Green Books and the Soil Association. Orderline is 01803 863260.
The Internet. Some useful websites are:
www.organicsdirect.com (fruit, vegetables, bread, wine, etc. available).
www.freshfood.co.uk (various quality foods available)
www.realmeat.co.uk (quality meats)
www.welsh-organic-meat.co.uk (meat, poultry, etc.)

APPENDIX 4

Diet Diary to Fill In

Use these blank charts to help you monitor your diet on the Freeform plan (see page 122). Just tick off each unit (or half unit in the case of Oil, Quality Carb and Calcium) as you use it and write in the meal spaces what you eat for each meal and snack. The six spaces for water each represent one glassful.

Units	Used	Meals
Protein		Breakfast
Oil		
Nut		Midmorning snack
Seed		Lunch
C-Fruit		
Fruit-2		
Green		Afternoon snack
Flame		
Pulse		Evening meal
Quality Carb		
Calcium		
Water	1	2	3	4	5	6

Units	Used	Meals
Protein		Breakfast
Oil		
Nut		Midmorning snack
Seed		Lunch
C-Fruit		
Fruit-2		
Green		Afternoon snack
Flame		
Pulse		Evening meal
Quality Carb		
Calcium		
Water	1	2	3	4	5	6

Units	Used	Meals
Protein		Breakfast
Oil	⟋	
Nut		Midmorning snack
Seed		
C-Fruit		Lunch
Fruit-2		
Green		Afternoon snack
Flame		
Pulse		Evening meal
Quality Carb	⟋	
Calcium	⟋	
Water	1	2	3	4	5	6

Units	Used	Meals
Protein		Breakfast
Oil	⟋	
Nut		Midmorning snack
Seed		
C-Fruit		Lunch
Fruit-2		
Green		Afternoon snack
Flame		
Pulse		Evening meal
Quality Carb	⟋	
Calcium	⟋	
Water	1	2	3	4	5	6

Units	Used	Meals				
Protein		Breakfast				
Oil						
Nut		Midmorning snack				
Seed		Lunch				
C-Fruit						
Fruit-2						
Green		Afternoon snack				
Flame						
Pulse		Evening meal				
Quality Carb						
Calcium						
Water	1	2	3	4	5	6

Units	Used	Meals				
Protein		Breakfast				
Oil						
Nut		Midmorning snack				
Seed		Lunch				
C-Fruit						
Fruit-2						
Green		Afternoon snack				
Flame						
Pulse		Evening meal				
Quality Carb						
Calcium						
Water	1	2	3	4	5	6

Units	Used	Meals				
Protein		Breakfast				
Oil	⟋					
Nut		Midmorning snack				
Seed		Lunch				
C-Fruit						
Fruit-2						
Green		Afternoon snack				
Flame						
Pulse		Evening meal				
Quality Carb	⟋					
Calcium	⟋					
Water	1	2	3	4	5	6

Units	Used	Meals				
Protein		Breakfast				
Oil	⟋					
Nut		Midmorning snack				
Seed		Lunch				
C-Fruit						
Fruit-2						
Green		Afternoon snack				
Flame						
Pulse		Evening meal				
Quality Carb	⟋					
Calcium	⟋					
Water	1	2	3	4	5	6

APPENDIX 5

Quick Guide to the Omega Units

Keep handy for reference

 PROTEIN UNIT Medium portion oily fish, large portion white fish, medium portion seafood, small portion organic lean meat, game, poultry or Quorn.

NOTE: One to two 1,000mg omega-3 fish oil capsules are obligatory with each Protein Unit except oily fish.

 OIL UNIT Two tablespoons of oil a day. Either plain, good quality olive oil (preferred choice for high-temperature cooking), or the oil blend – olive oil blended with rapeseed oil (ratio of 100ml olive oil to 75ml rapeseed oil) for other cooking, or salad oil blend – a blend of one-third each rapeseed, walnut and groundnut oil for salads and cold use. The Oil Unit can be divided into two portions, used separately.

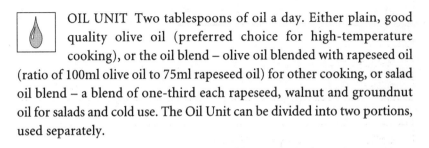 NUT UNIT Your unit is an average palmful. It will usually be a mix of fresh nuts in the ratio of 50% walnuts, 25% cashews and 25% hazelnuts. If nut mix is stated, use this. Occasionally within the 14-day diet other nuts are specified.

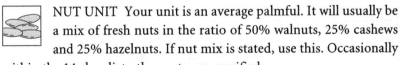 SEED UNIT One heaped tablespoon seed mix, which is in the ratio of 50% pumpkin seeds, 25% linseeds and 25% sunflower seeds. If seed mix is stated, use this. Occasionally within the 14-day diet other seeds are specified.

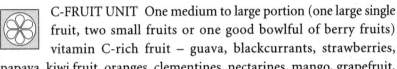 C-FRUIT UNIT One medium to large portion (one large single fruit, two small fruits or one good bowlful of berry fruits) vitamin C-rich fruit – guava, blackcurrants, strawberries, papaya, kiwi fruit, oranges, clementines, nectarines, mango, grapefruit, raspberries or a mixture of any of these. Eat raw.

FRUIT-2 UNIT One medium to large portion of any other fresh fruit – apples, peaches, melon, cherries, red grapes, plums, pears (preferred choices). Mostly raw. Choose other fruits from time to time if you like (such as bananas).

OR one small to medium portion dried fruits – apricots, prunes, figs (preferred choices). Choose raisins and sultanas from time to time if you like. You can use them ready to eat or re-constituted without added sugar.

GREEN UNIT One portion or two smaller portions (or more) of any fresh mid to dark green vegetable or mixture of these – kale, spring greens, savoy or other dark cabbage, sprouts, spinach, green beans, broccoli (calabrese), purple sprouting broccoli, seaweed (preferred choices). Other choices are green beans, cos or other dark lettuce, mangetout and peas.

FLAME UNIT One medium to large portion of any fresh red, orange or yellow vegetable – red peppers, orange peppers, yellow peppers, tomatoes, carrots, orange-fleshed squash or pumpkin, swede, sweetcorn or a mixture of these.

PULSE UNIT One medium portion (about 150g cooked weight) pulses – dried beans, peas or lentils, such as Puy lentils, green lentils, kidney beans, cannellini beans, borlotti beans, butter beans, broad beans, baked beans, chickpeas, split peas, soya protein products such as tofu or TVP, lentil paté or hummus.

QUALITY CARB UNIT This can be any one of the following.

○ Up to 80g (about three slices) any wholegrain bread or one large wholewheat pitta or chapati.
○ Up to four plain oatcakes or six dark rye crispbreads (such as Ryvita).
○ One good portion (about 60g dry weight) wholegrain, such as brown basmati rice, wholewheat pasta, bulghar wheat, pot barley, oats, buckwheat, quinoa, millet or amaranth.

- One good portion (about 60g) wholegrain breakfast cereal, such as shredded wheat, old-fashioned porridge, All-Bran, muesli (the kind with no added sugar or salt), puffed wheat or Weetabix.
- One good portion (about 225g) new potatoes in their skins.
- One medium orange-fleshed sweet potato.
- OR 2 × half portions of any of these.

 CALCIUM UNIT At least 200g low-fat natural bio yogurt or calcium-enriched soya yogurt OR at least 300ml skimmed milk or calcium-enriched soya milk.

OR 2 × half portions of any of these.

Small tub of low-fat fromage frais, cottage cheese or half-fat Greek yogurt can be used occasionally.

 WATER UNIT Six to eight 8 to 10fl oz (225ml to 300ml) glasses of water a day, spaced out evenly. Before, with or just after meals or when exercising is ideal. See unlimiteds (page 105) for what you can add to this.

INDEX